A Color Atlas of
E.N.T. Diagnosis

A Color Atlas of

E. N. T.
Diagnosis

Revised 2nd Edition

T.R. Bull FRCS

Consultant Surgeon
Royal National Throat Nose and Ear Hospital, London
Senior Lecturer to the Institute of Laryngology & Otology
Consultant Surgeon, Charing Cross Hospital, London

Provided as a service

by
Merrell Dow U.S.A.

Copyright © T. R. Bull, 1974, 1987
Second edition published by Wolfe Medical Publications Ltd, 1987

Printed by W.S. Cowell Ltd, Buttermarket, Ipswich, England
ISBN 0 72340894 7 cased edition
ISBN 0 72340923 4 limp edition

General Editor, Wolfe Medical Atlases: G. Barry Carruthers,
MD(London)

Introduction

It is over 10 years since the first Color Atlas of ENT Diagnosis was published and it is gratifying that it has appeared also in several other languages. The presentation and pattern of disease alters little in a decade and new diagnoses or recognition of new diseases are few. Nonetheless, ideas change, investigations improve and advances are made. These factors, therefore, together with shortcomings pointed out in reviews of previous editions, call for an updated and hopefully improved Atlas.

Fibreoptic instruments become more established for use in endoscopy of the upper respiratory tract. Panoramic photographs of hitherto poorly seen sites such as the post-nasal space are now obtainable. Wide view pictures of the ear drum and meatus can be achieved with fibreoptic techniques. Such a clear and obvious presentation of the pathology is not seen, however, in routine practice and although some of these pictures have been included in this Atlas, they have not been emphasised.

The format of the book is unaltered and I have tried to keep the text succinct without discussion of varying opinions. The more obvious, but not gross examples of various disorders have been selected in the hope that the color photographs will continue to serve as a practical help in diagnosis. There may still be a bias to those conditions that lend themselves to photography. Brief details of medical and surgical treatment where useful and of interest are also included. This new edition of the Atlas, I hope, will continue to stimulate an interest in ear, nose and throat conditions for medical students and will be useful for those in general practice, casualty and those training in ENT surgery or allied specialities. The basic structure remains, without radical changes, as an introduction to ear, nose and throat surgery and an adjunct to the standard larger texts.

Contents

Acknowledgements

I wish to thank Mr Martin Bailey, my colleague at the Royal National Throat Nose and Ear Hospital and Dr Tony Steel, my general practitioner for their advice on the text and content of the book. Most of the photographs were taken by myself but I am grateful for the expertise of the Photographic Department at the Royal National Throat Nose and Ear Hospital for many of the better illustrations. My thanks also to Mr Tony Cheesman (**396**), Dr Alec Davies (**102**), Mr John Evans (**366**), Mr Graham Frazer (**23/24/25**), Dr Glyn Lloyd (**27**), Dr Reck (**52/53/145**), Mr Charles Smith (**142**) and Mr Valentine Hammond (**118**) for contributing these pictures.

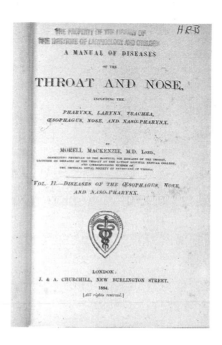

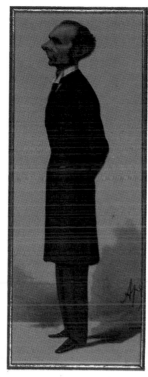

The frontispiece and two volumes of Morrell MacKenzie's first standard text book on Rhinology and Laryngology.

Sir Morrell MacKenzie

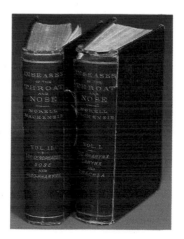

THIS CARTOON drawn in 1887 shows the austere Scottish physician and surgeon, who founded Ear, Nose and Throat as a speciality and wrote the first standard textbook on Rhinology and Laryngology. Sir Morrell MacKenzie also founded one of the first hospitals for Nose and Throat diseases in London in 1863 (today, the Royal National Throat Nose and Ear Hospital). The most common condition he treated in this hospital was laryngeal tuberculosis, at that time invariably fatal, and today rare and curable.

Examination

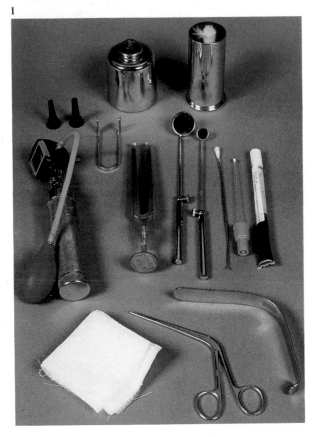

1 The instruments needed for an ENT examination The **head mirror** (**2**) gives effective lighting for examining the upper respiratory tract and ear, and leaves both hands free for using instruments. Initially, the technique of using a head mirror is not easy, and some may prefer a *fibreoptic* or electric *headlight* (**3**).

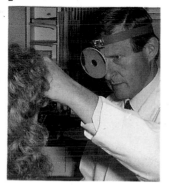

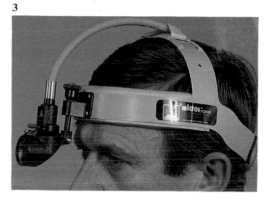

The **laryngeal and post-nasal mirrors** require warming to avoid misting, and hot water or a spirit lamp is necessary.

An angled **tongue depressor** or wooden spatula is needed for examining the oropharynx and post-nasal space.

Angled forceps are used for dressing the nose or ear.

A **tuning fork** is essential for the diagnosis of conductive or sensorineural (perceptive) hearing loss. A C_1 or C_2 (256 or 512 cps) is needed. The very large tuning forks used to test vibration sense are unsatisfactory and may give a false Rinne test.

A **Jobson-Horne probe** is widely used in ENT departments: a loop on one end is for removing wax (and foreign bodies) from the ear or nose. Cotton wool attached to the other end is used for cleaning the ear.

An **auriscope, nasal and aural specula** complete the basic instruments.

A sterile swab and media is necessary for throat, nasal or ear specimens to be taken for culture and sensitivity. A 'narrow' swab holder as shown here is extremely useful for aural specimens, for the more common swab is too wide and traumatic for the deep meatus and middle ear.

Examination of the ear

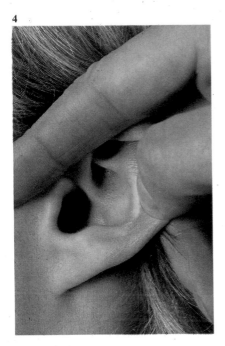 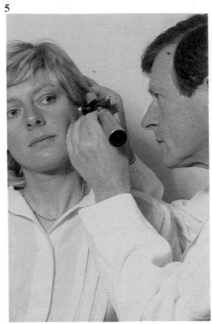

4   Retracting the pinna The meatus is tortuous: to see the drum the pinna is therefore retracted backwards and outwards, and the index finger may be used to hold the tragus forward.

5   The auriscope This is best held like a pen. In this way, the examiner's little finger can rest on the patient's cheek; if the patient's head moves, the position of the ear speculum is maintained in the meatus.

6

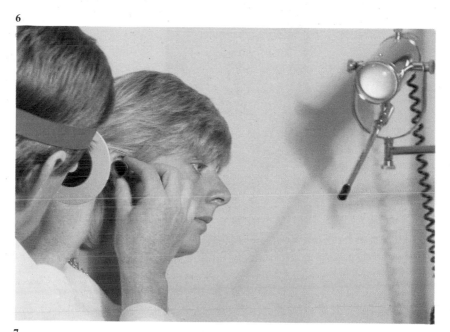

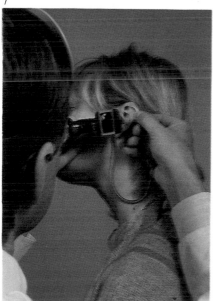

6 Head mirror and speculum These are used for the initial examination of the meatus and drum.

7 A pneumatic otoscope A hand-held air filled bulb attached to the auriscope enables air to be gently inflated against the drum demonstrating drum mobility. Reduced mobility is conspicuous and diagnostic of middle ear fluid. Reduced mobility is also seen with a drum that may be of a normal appearance but in which there is malleus fixation, or with tympanosclerosis.

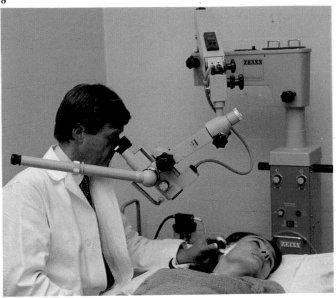

9

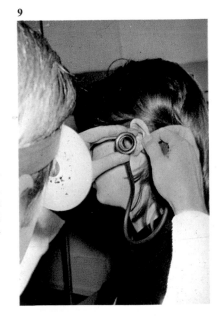

8 Microscope examination of the drum Although most drums can be seen well and conditions diagnosed with the auriscope, the increased magnification that is obtainable with the operating microscope is sometimes necessary, and this apparatus is standard for a well-equipped out-patient department.

9 Siegle's speculum has been displaced by the pneumatic otoscope, but Siegle's speculum with *plain* non-magnifying glass is *very* useful to test drum mobility with the microscope.

10 A normal drum The main landmarks seen on the pars tensa of a normal drum are the lateral process (*top arrow*) and handle (*middle arrow*) of the malleus and the light reflex (*lower arrow*). The drum superior to the short process is the pars flaccida or attic part of the drum. A normal drum is grey and varies in vascularity and translucency.

11 A more vascular drum with vessels extending down the handle of the malleus to the umbo.

12 The **incus** may show as a shadow through a thin drum, as may less commonly the round window and opening of the Eustachian tube.

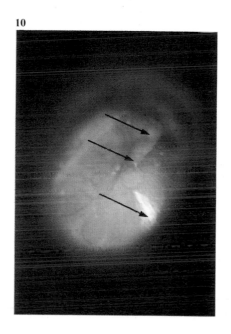

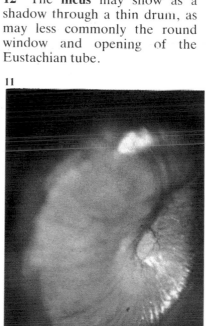

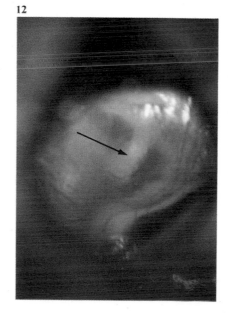

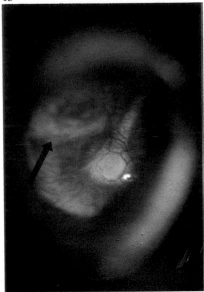

13 The chorda tympani nerve

The chorda tympani is the nerve of taste to the anterior two-thirds of the tongue (excluding the circumvallate papillae), and is also secretomotor nerve to the submandibular and sublingual salivary glands. The chorda tympani usually lies behind the pars flaccida and is not visible, but if the nerve is more inferior it shows through the drum.

If examination of the drum and meatus is normal in a patient complaining of earache, the pain is **referred**. **Referred otalgia** may be from nearby structures such as the temporo-mandibular joint, neck muscles or cervical spine; it may be from the teeth, tongue, tonsils or larynx. The Vth, IXth and Xth cranial nerves which supply these sites have their respective tympanic and auricular branches supplying the ear. Earache also frequently precedes a Bell's palsy.

Hearing loss

14   Conductive and sensori-neural (perceptive) hearing loss   Hearing loss is either conductive or sensori-neural in type: it is an essential basic step in diagnosis of hearing loss to distinguish between these two. Sensori-neural hearing loss is either due to a cochlear or retro-cochlear lesion.

Most hearing loss is easy to diagnose into a well-defined conductive or sensori-neural type. ('Mixed' hearing loss may occur but this diagnosis is usually non-contributory and the term is better avoided.)

Lesions to the left of the blue line cause conductive hearing loss, and are frequently curable: hearing loss to the right of the blue line is due to a sensori-neural lesion and is usually not so amenable to treatment.

14

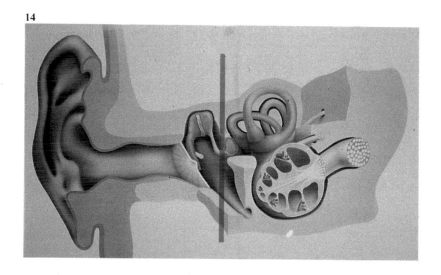

15

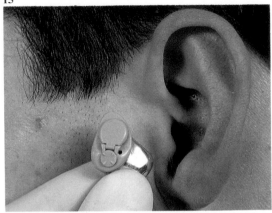

16

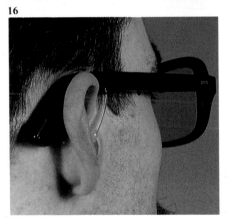

17

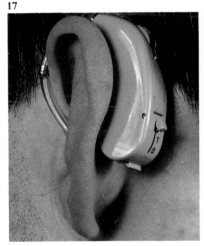

15,16,17 Modern **hearing aids**

Conductive hearing loss that is not amenable to surgical treatment responds well to conventional hearing aids, as may sensori-neural hearing loss with a 'flat' tracing in which the hearing loss is equal at most frequencies. Most commonly, however, sensori-neural hearing loss affects the high tones, with relatively good hearing at the low frequencies. The problems with hearing aids to achieve good speech discrimination for this type of hearing loss still present difficulties. Aids, which contain a microphone, amplifier, battery and earphone, can be fitted either behind the ear, or to spectacles or, in certain cases, with an in-the-ear aid.

Tests for conductive and sensori-neural hearing loss

18

19

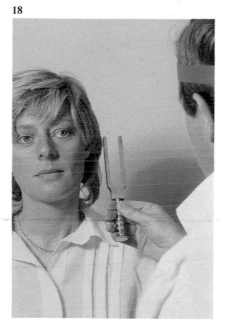
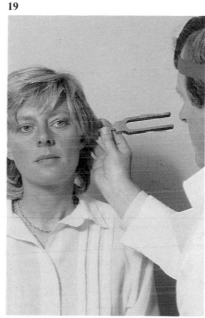

18, 19   The Rinne test The tuning fork tests are essential preliminary tests for the diagnosis of hearing loss. The Rinne and Weber tests enable the diagnosis of a conductive or sensori-neural hearing loss to be made. If the tuning fork is heard louder on the mastoid process than in front of the ear, the Rinne is negative and the hearing loss is conductive. If the tuning fork is heard better in front of the ear, the Rinne is positive and the hearing is either normal or there is a sensori-neural hearing loss.

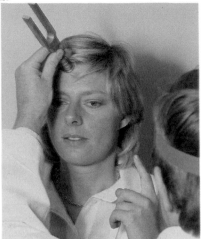 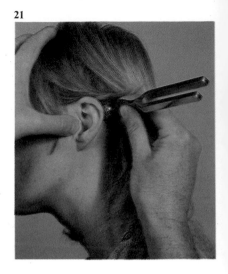

20 The Weber test The tuning fork when held in the midline on the forehead is heard in the ear with the conductive hearing loss. This test is very sensitive and if the meatus is occluded with the finger, the tuning fork is heard in that ear. A conductive loss of as little as five decibels will result in the Weber being referred to that ear.

21 The occlusion test (Bing) is also helpful. The tuning fork is held on the mastoid process and the tragus lightly pushed to occlude the meatus. The tuning fork is heard louder. In conductive hearing loss, even of a slight degree, there is no change when the meatus is occluded. The Rinne test does not become negative until there is a marked degree of conductive loss (about a 20 decibel air-bone gap). It is therefore possible to have a slight conductive hearing loss with a positive Rinne. The more sensitive occlusion test will help in the diagnosis.

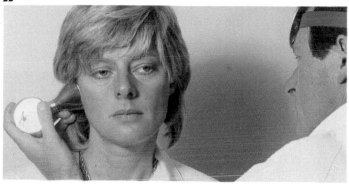

Total hearing loss in one ear is frequently wrongly diagnosed as a conductive hearing loss. The Rinne is negative, because the tuning fork, although not heard in front of the ear, when placed on the mastoid process of the deaf ear, is heard by the better ear, the sound being transmitted by the bone (false negative Rinne). The Weber should give the clue that the Rinne is false, for it will not lateralise to the deaf ear.

22 Barany box This is used to confirm the diagnosis of total hearing loss. It is placed on the good ear and produces a noise totally masking this ear. The patient will be unable to repeat words clearly spoken into the deaf ear.

Total hearing loss in one ear may be congenital or result from a skull fracture. Meningitis is also a cause, but *mumps* is probably the commonest cause of this type of hearing loss. An acoustic neuroma may present with a unilateral sensori-neural loss, frequently total. If this type of deafness is associated with a canal paresis on the caloric test, and an enlarged internal auditory meatus on X-ray, an acoustic tumour is probable. These are basic preliminary tests in the diagnosis of early acoustic neuromas.

23

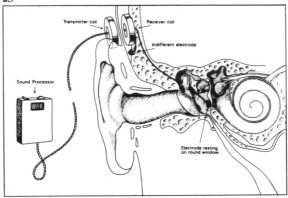

SINGLE CHANNEL
ROUND WINDOW IMPLANT
IN POSITION

24

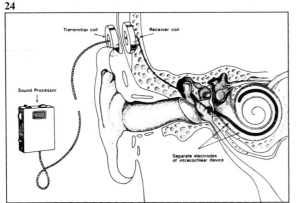

MULTICHANNEL
INTRACOCHLEAR IMPLANT
IN POSITION

25

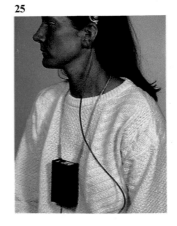

23,24,25 *Total hearing loss involving both ears* has stimulated innovative surgery in the last decade to develop an electronic *cochlear implant*. At present, techniques achieve some appreciation of sound to those previously totally deaf.

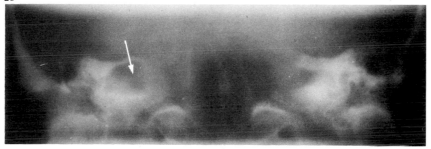

26 Acoustic neuroma A unilateral sensori-neural hearing loss may be caused by an acoustic neuroma. The hearing loss is often profound or total. In the past, when the hearing loss was ignored acoustic neuromas were not infrequently diagnosed late when they were large with other more obvious symptoms and signs of a space occupying intra-cranial lesion. There is now a marked awareness that sensori-neural hearing loss, particularly if unilateral, requires investigation to exclude an early acoustic neuroma. Polytomogram X-rays of the internal auditory meatus (associated with an absent or impaired caloric response—see page 33) represent the most helpful preliminary investigation in the diagnosis of an acoustic neuroma. *Arrow* indicates the enlarged internal auditory meatus.

27 Two important X ray innovations developed in Great Britain in the past decade are **CT scan** (computerised tomography) and **NMR** (nuclear magnetic resonance) — termed *MRI* (magnetic resonance imaging) in USA. The CT scan and NMR tomograms have many useful applications in head and neck radiology and are very helpful in the diagnosis of acoustic neuromas (*arrow*).

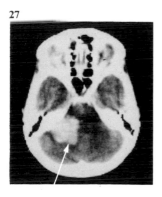

Investigation of hearing loss

28 Audiometry *A pure tone audiogram* is the standard test of hearing level. The readings are recorded on a chart with intensity (0 – 100 decibels) and frequency (usually 250–8000 cps). A normal tracing is between −10dB and +10dB at all frequencies. This test is accurate to about 10 decibels only for there are variables in the patient's responses, and the audiometrician and the machine's accuracy. Hearing is tested in front of the ear (air conduction—recorded in black) and over the mastoid process (bone conduction—in red).

A silent or sound-proof room is necessary for accurate pure tone audiometry.

29 Audiograms The one on the left shows a typical sensori-neural hearing loss: a sharp dip at 4000 cps as on this chart is typical of inner ear damage due to *noise trauma*. A loss of high frequencies is commonly seen in senile hearing loss—*presbycusis*.

The audiogram on the right shows a conductive hearing loss with the sound heard better on the bone, typical of *otosclerosis*, or *otitis media*.

Audiometry requires skill and training, particularly to test children. An audiogram is obtainable from most children by the age of 3–4 years. With unilateral hearing loss, noise is used to mask the better ear, so that this ear does not hear the sound transmission from the deaf ear and give a false reading. Hearing assessment under the age of 3 years, or in children who are unable to cooperate with audiometry, requires special skills and techniques. Response of a baby or toddler to meaningful sounds, such as a spoon 'chinked' against a cup, gives an. indication of hearing. **Electrocochleography** involves placing fine electrodes through the drum to pick up auditory nerve reaction potential in response to sound. This refined test gives a good hearing assessment in infants in whom a hearing loss is suspected. Anaesthesia is required for electrocochleography (Ecog): this objective test of hearing acuity is also of help in the diagnosis of psychosomatic hearing loss or malingering. The auditory brain stem response in which electroencephalogram recordings are made following auditory stimulus is another useful audiometric test.

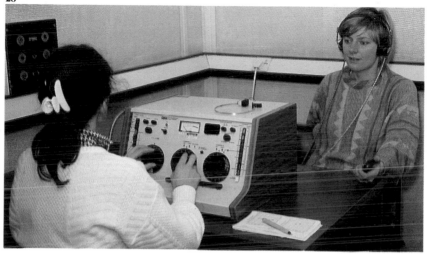

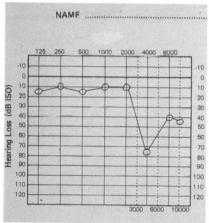

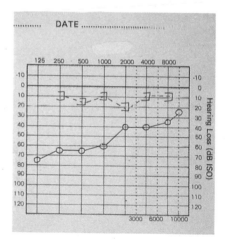

SPEECH AUDIOGRAM

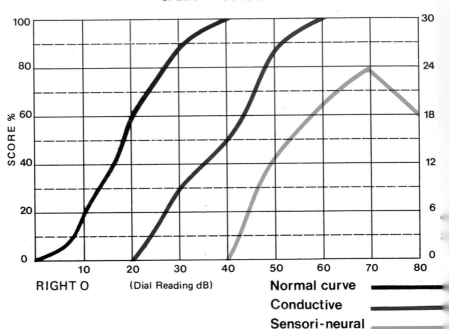

RIGHT O   (Dial Reading dB)

Normal curve ▬▬▬
Conductive ▬▬▬
Sensori-neural ▬▬▬

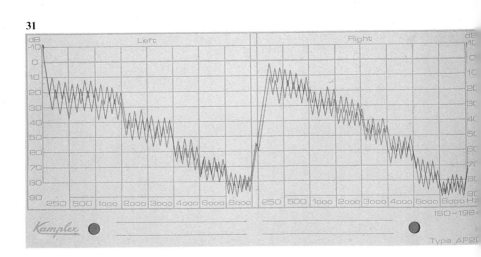

30 Speech discrimination audiometry A criticism of pure tone audiometry is that an assessment of the ability to hear pure tone sounds may not reflect the ability to hear speech. A phonetically balanced list of words is used. The percentage of those correctly detected is used as the index to plot a speech discrimination chart.

The ability to understand speech is obviously reduced with all hearing loss but particularly with sensori-neural loss in which the high tones are involved. An additional help in the diagnosis of acoustic neuromas may be extremely poor speech discrimination, in excess of that expected from the level of the pure tone or Bekesy audiogram.

31 Bekesy audiometry This gives a more complete and accurate test of hearing than a pure tone audiogram. The response to both interrupted and continuous sound over a wide range of frequencies is recorded. Certain patterns of tracing are associated with types of sensori-neural hearing loss, which help in diagnosis. It is sometimes possible to distinguish cochlear from retrocochlear hearing loss and this is an important investigation for acoustic neuroma. This audiogram shows a high tone hearing loss due to presbycusis. With retrocochlear lesions, hearing for continuous sound fatigues and the tracing therefore separates from that of interrupted sound.

32

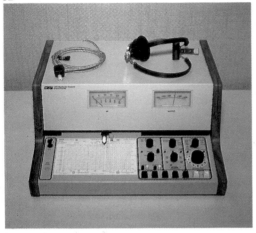

32, 33 Impedance audiometry This involves several measurements giving a wide range of information about the middle and inner ear. A probe with a rubber tip and containing three small patent tubes is fitted into the meatus to make an airtight seal. One tube delivers the tone to the ear, one is attached to a microphone to monitor the sound pressure level within the ear canal, and the third is attached to a manometer to vary the air pressure in the ear. The measurements are particularly helpful in the differential diagnosis of conductive and sensori-neural hearing losses, giving information about middle ear pressure, Eustachian tube function, middle ear reflexes, and the level of a lower motor neurone facial nerve palsy. It is now widely used to confirm the presence of middle ear fluid, and the 'flat' tracing is characteristic. A 'glue ear' may be diagnosed in children under the age of 3½-4 years with impedance measurements when cooperation for a pure tone is not possible.

33

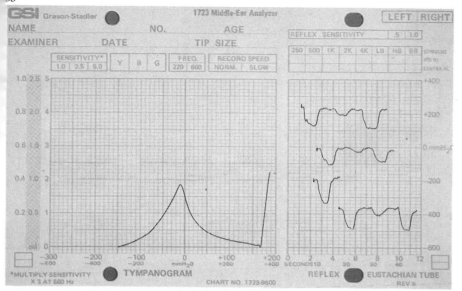

Tests of balance

Vertigo is most commonly due to a disorder of the labyrinth. A sensation of unsteadiness may occur, however, with hypoglycaemia, orthostatic hypotension, hyperventilation and cerebral ischaemia; tumours or multiple sclerosis involving the vestibular system also cause imbalance.

34

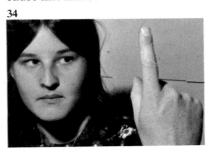

34 Observation for nystagmus is one of the clinical tests for abnormalities of balance. Nystagmus due to a labyrinth disorder is characterised by a slow and quick phase of eye movement: the eye moves slowly away from the side of the involved labyrinth, and flicks rapidly back to that side; the nystagmus is said to be in the direction of the quick phase. The eye movement in nystagmus is fine, and observation of this sign is facilitated if the patient is fitted with glasses with magnifying lenses—**Frenzel glasses (35)**.

35

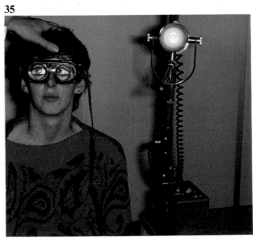

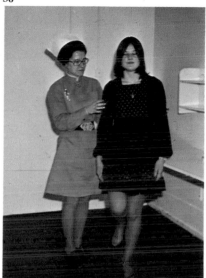 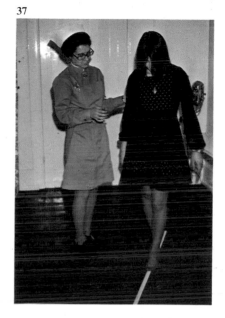

36 The Romberg test is another basic test of balance. This test, in which the patient is asked to stand still with feet together and eyes closed, is made more sensitive by asking the patient to mark time.

37 Tests to demonstrate abnormalities of gait One of these is heel toe walking along a straight line: a person with normal balance is stable without looking down at the feet.

Abnormalities in these preliminary clinical tests of balance will indicate the need for further investigation.

Vertigo due to a labyrinth disorder may occur with or without hearing loss.

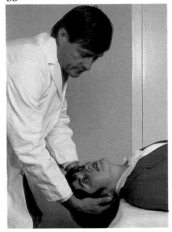

38   Positional vertigo *Benign paroxysmal positional vertigo* is a sudden and severe rotary vertigo occurring on lying down in bed, or on looking upwards, when the head is placed backwards and to one side. There is no hearing loss, and it may follow a head injury. Although common, it is frequently not recognised and unnecessary neurological investigation may be carried out.

The positional history is typical, and diagnosis is confirmed by a positive positional test: when the head is placed backwards and to one side, nystagmus fatigues within several seconds but recurs temporarily when the patient sits up.

This is a self-limiting condition and simply avoiding the position that triggers off the attack may suffice as treatment. Positional vertigo may also occur with space occupying lesions involving the cerebellum and cerebello-pontine angle. Nystagmus may be induced with the positional test, but there is no latent period and the nystagmus does not fatigue.

39 Vertebro-basilar ischaemia
Vertigo with head movement, or transient sudden loss of consciousness ('drop' attacks), occur with temporary interruption of the blood supply to the labyrinth or cerebral cortex. This condition is seen in the older age group with cervical osteoarthritis, and with evidence of hypertension and atherosclerosis. Movement of the irregular cervical spine temporarily occludes the tortuous atherosclerotic vertebral vessels which lead to the basilar and internal auditory arteries.

This *vertebral angiogram* shows the kinking of the vertebral artery.

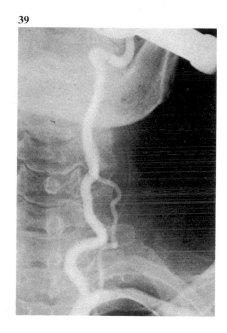

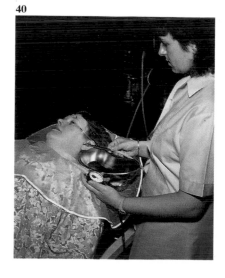

40 The caloric test Irrigation of the external meatus with water 7° above and later 7° below body temperature sets up convection currents of the endolymph in the semicircular canals. This causes nystagmus and the duration of the nystagmus gives an index of the activity of the labyrinth. The nystagmus can be directly observed or recorded electrically (*electronystagmography*). This test is particularly valuable in the diagnosis of Meniere's disease and acoustic neuroma. A reduced or absent nystagmus is found (canal paresis).

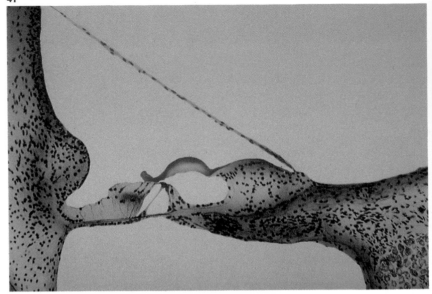

41, 42 Meniere's disease *Sudden severe rotary vertigo* often with nausea and vomiting, a *tinnitus* increasing prior to the vertigo, and a *sensori-neural hearing loss* (cochlear type) form the triad of symptoms characteristic of *Meniere's disease*. In this curious condition there is an increase in the endolymph volume, but the cause is unknown. The disease has a reputation for being serious which is not justified. Although the vertigo may occasionally be severe and incapacitating, the symptoms are frequently mild, usually self-limiting and not progressive. It is never fatal, and medical treatment with labyrinthine sedatives eg prochlorperazine (Stemetil) commonly control the vertigo. Oral histamine-like drugs which aim to increase the blood flow to the inner ear (eg Serc) may also be effective but there is no proven specific medical therapy at present available for Meniere's. Many innovative surgical procedures have been tried: none has proved totally successful although decompression of the endolymphatic sac in an attempt to reduce the pressure in the scala media is the present favoured conservative surgery. Surgery to destroy the labyrinth is effective in controlling the vertigo but an irreversible total hearing loss, with an accentuated tinnitus are among the factors that make this treatment a last resort.

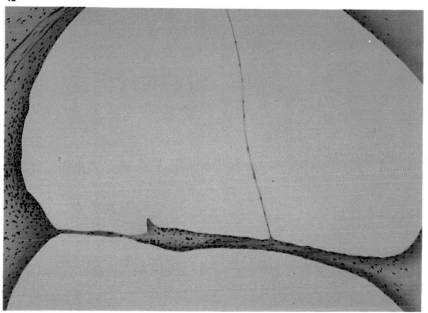

Tinnitus is commonly associated with hearing loss (although it may rarely be troublesome with normal hearing). The tinnitus with conductive hearing loss is usually less distressing than that with sensorineural hearing loss where the tinnitus may cause serious psychiatric disturbance. The full physiology and pathology of tinnitus remains unknown. There is no entirely effective treatment for tinnitus. Explanation and reassurance are helpful in the patient's acceptance of tinnitus (patients frequently associate it with serious intracranial disease) and the use of a tranquilliser may be necessary. *Tinnitus-maskers* in which a hearing aid-like device feeds a noise that has been matched with the tinnitus into the ear, may mask the tinnitus to a greater or lesser degree and be effective treatment. Surgical treatment of tinnitus with section of the acoustic nerve or destruction of the inner ear has been tried and is unsatisfactory.

Examination of the nose

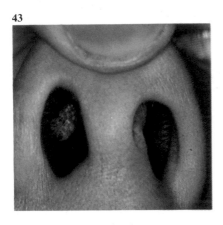

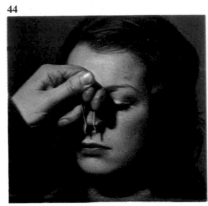

43 Examining a child Instruments are best avoided in children: a good view of the nose anteriorly can be obtained simply by pressing on the tip of the nose. In this case a clear view is obtained of a pedunculated papilloma.

44 A nasal speculum is needed to see more posteriorly. There are several different types of nasal speculum used throughout the world. (The one demonstrated here is the Thudicum speculum.)

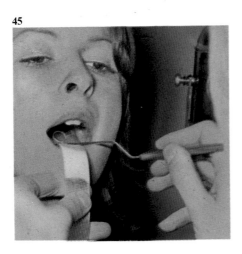

45 The post-nasal space is not easy to examine, particularly in children. With a patient who gags easily, or whose soft palate is close to the posterior wall of the oropharynx, a view may be impossible.

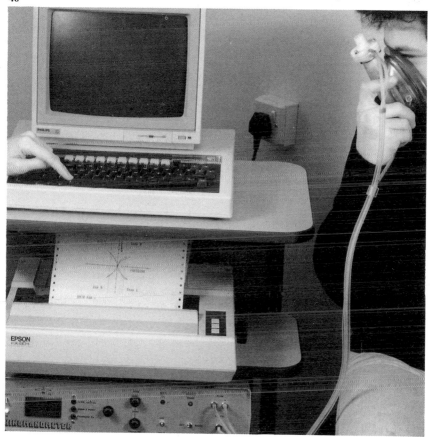

46 Rhinomanometry techniques give a *quantitative* measurement of nasal airway. Many methods have been employed but the anterior active method has gained most acceptance. The pressure is measured through one nostril, while the flow is measured through the opposite side using a facemask and pneumotach. Rhinomanometry has yet to become of sufficient clinical value to be of routine use in the assessment of nasal obstruction.

Sinus X-rays and transillumination

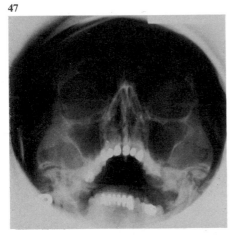

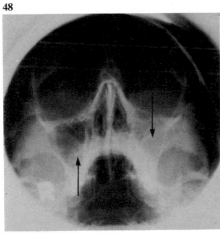

47,48,49 X-ray showing maxillary sinuses The sinus most commonly involved in disease is the maxillary sinus. An X-ray will show opacity (**48**, *top arrow*) suggesting infection or polyposis, or opacity with bone destruction suggestive of a neoplasm. The polypoid swelling (shown here in the floor of the left antrum, **48**, *lower arrow*), or thickening of the antral mucosa (**49**, *arrow*) are frequent chance findings, and in the absence of symptoms or other signs are probably not significant. A straight anterior-posterior X-ray shows the ethmoid and frontal sinuses, and a lateral and base of skull view shows the sphenoid sinus.

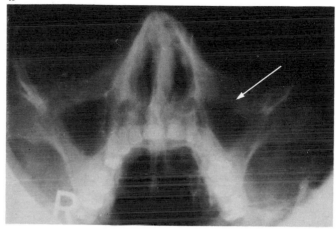

50 Transillumination A bright light held inside the mouth in a dark room is an investigation seldom used now that sinus X-rays are readily available. A dull antrum is however an additional sign in the diagnosis of maxillary sinus disease. Transillumination is useful to assess whether a sinusitis is settling. Dental cysts involving the antrum transilluminate brightly.

50

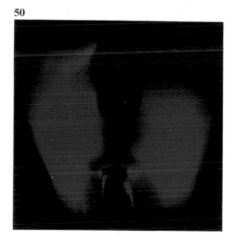

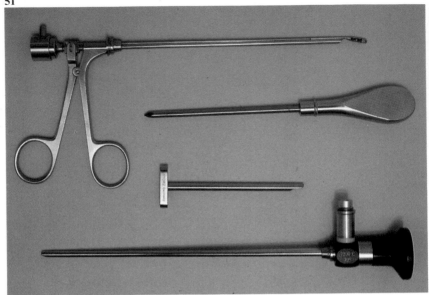

51,52 Sinus endoscopy (antroscopy) A narrow endoscope inserted into the maxillary antrum, either through the thin bony wall of the canine fossa intra-orally, or via the inferior meatus of the nasal fossa under the inferior turbinate, gives a good view of the interior of the maxillary sinus and is helpful in diagnosis. There is a noticeable loss of vocal resonance with nasal obstruction, but this is a very conspicuous sign when the maxillary antra are filled with fluid. In the same way that fluid in the lung, for which the well-known change of sound on auscultation is diagnostic, a stethoscope held over the maxillary sinus will detect a similar alteration in sound transmission. **Diagnostic ultrasound techniques** have made use of this, and instruments are now available in which ultrasonic waves are directed into the antrum, and reflect differently when the sinus contains fluid. Ultrasound for the diagnosis of maxillary sinusitis has not become established and standard sinus X-rays remain a more reliable help in the diagnosis of sinusitis.

52

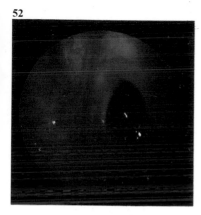

52   The ostium of the maxillary sinus as seen through the endoscope.

53

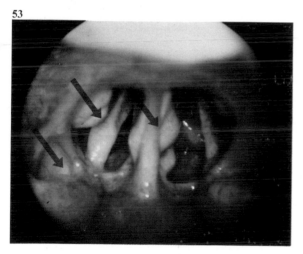

53   **The post-nasal space** A panoramic view showing most of the anatomical features photographed through the fibreoptic endoscope (see **58**). (*Left arrow*—Eustachian orifice; *middle arrow*—posterior end of inferior turbinate; *right arrow*—posterior border of septum.)

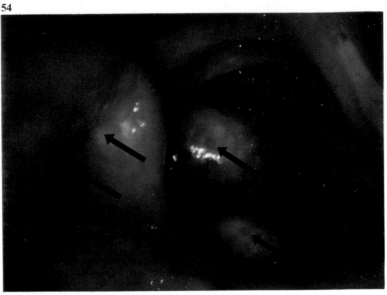

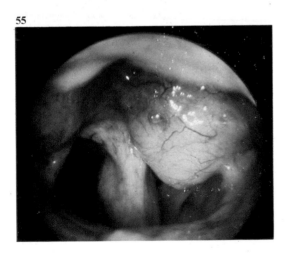

54 **The post-nasal space** Enlarged view of **53** to show the Eustachian orifice and posterior ends of the middle and inferior turbinate.

55 A post-nasal cyst (Thornvaldts) demonstrated with a fibreoptic photograph of the post-nasal space.

Examining the pharynx and larynx

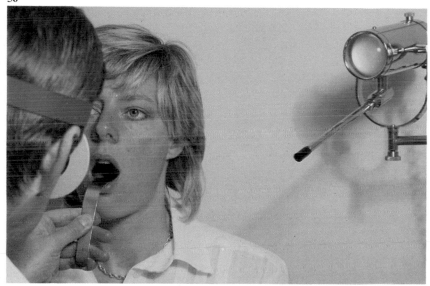

56 Examination of the pharynx A tongue depressor is necessary to obtain a clear view of the tonsillar region.

57

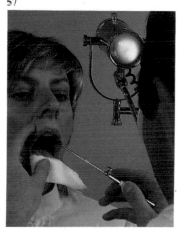

57 Examination of the larynx using the laryngeal mirror (indirect laryngoscopy) A good view of the larynx is easily obtained with most patients: the valleculae, pyriform fossae, arytenoids, ventricular bands and cords should all be clearly seen. It requires some inhibition of the gag reflex by the patient, and a local anaesthetic lozenge or spray may be necessary. The tongue is held between the thumb and middle finger and the upper lip retracted with the index finger. This examination is difficult in children not only because they may be uncooperative, but because the infantile epiglottis is curved, unlike the 'flat' adult epiglottis, and occludes a clear view of the larynx. Direct laryngoscopy under anaesthetic is usually necessary, therefore, to diagnose the cause of hoarseness in a child. Fibreoptic instruments for laryngoscopy have recently been developed and are a further useful technique in seeing the larynxes of adults and children, which may be difficult on indirect examination.

58 Fibreoptic endoscopy of the upper respiratory tract When the post-nasal space and larynx are difficult to see with routine mirror examination, the development of a narrow fibreoptic tube, which can be inserted through the nose, gives a helpful view of the nasal fossae, post-nasal space (see **53,54,55**) and the larynx. A topical anaesthetic is used to the nasal mucosa before the endoscope is introduced. The field is small, however, and one has to be experienced in the use of the present fibreoptic endoscopes to be confident of excluding pathology in the larynx.

58

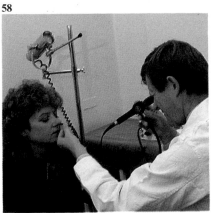

59

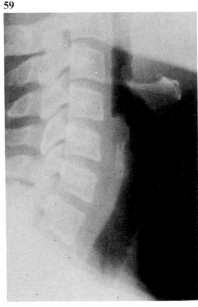

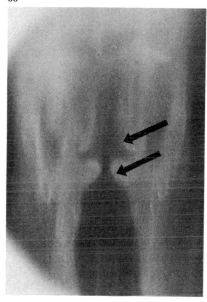

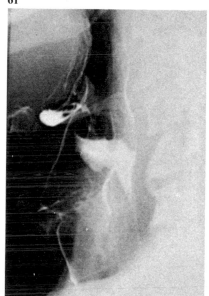

59 A lateral X-ray of the neck gives helpful information about the anatomy of the base of the tongue, larynx, trachea and upper oesophagus. The upper oesophagus is normally approximately the width of the trachea. An increase in the width of the oesophagus is very suggestive of significant pathology needing further investigation, such as a barium swallow X-ray or oesophagoscopy.

60 Laryngeal tomogram This shows the cords (*lower arrow*) and ventricular bands (*upper arrow*), and is used to confirm the site and extent of a lesion. Small lesions on the cord can be detected, and 'hidden sites' in the larynx such as the ventricle and subglottic region are well demonstrated.

61 Laryngogram Contrast medium X-rays of the larynx are little used. Although the anatomy is well shown, good pictures are technically difficult to achieve, and require a lot of patience by the subject and radiographer. Good tomograms have tended to displace the laryngogram as an investigation.

Taste and smell

62 Solutions used to test taste and smell Four solutions are used to test taste. The solution is placed on one side of the tongue and the patient asked to identify the taste, whether sweet, salt, sour or bitter. This is a relatively crude qualitative test.

Testing for anosmia is with a series of smell solutions for the patient to recognise.

62

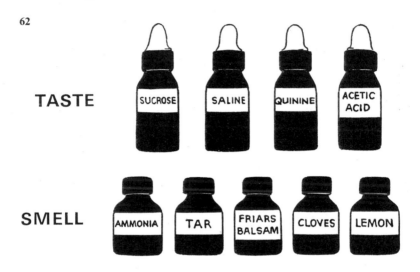

TASTE SUCROSE SALINE QUININE ACETIC ACID

SMELL AMMONIA TAR FRIARS BALSAM CLOVES LEMON

63 Anosmia 'scratch card' tests A more recent innovation is a disc impregnated with a specific odour which is released when the disc is scratched with the finger nail; the smell identity is marked on the card. Quantitative tests are not in routine clinical use, although 'olfactometers' with measured odours for smell assessment are described.

Anosmia may be a complication of fracture of the anterior cranial fossa, or it may follow influenza: recovery is uncommon. Temporary anosmia will occur with severe nasal obstruction. Anosmia is invariably linked with a complaint of impaired taste: taste is usually found to be normal on testing and the sensation of smell is an adjunct to the full subtle appreciation of taste. The dependence on smell for taste appreciation varies from person to person, so that a complaint of taste loss may or may not accompany anosmia.

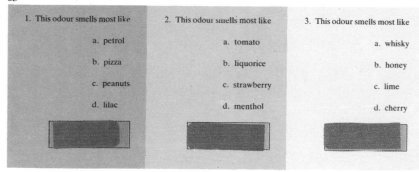

1. This odour smells most like	2. This odour smells most like	3. This odour smells most like
a. petrol	a. tomato	a. whisky
b. pizza	b. liquorice	b. honey
c. peanuts	c. strawberry	c. lime
d. lilac	d. menthol	d. cherry

One is dependent on the integrity of the patient's response to smell and taste tests. It is, therefore, often impossible to be certain in medicolegal cases whether anosmia or ageusia is genuine. With smell, a failure to identify a very strong stimulus such as ammonia suggests malingering, for the Vth and not the Ist cranial nerve is involved.

64 Electrogustometry Electricity has a metallic taste and when a small current in micro-amps is applied to the tongue, a quantitative reading can be obtained. The normal threshold on the margin of the tongue is between 5 and $30\mu a$. This more refined test of taste is of value in conditions such as facial palsy or acoustic neuromas in which the chorda tympani nerve may be involved.

64

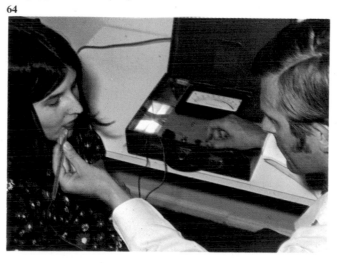

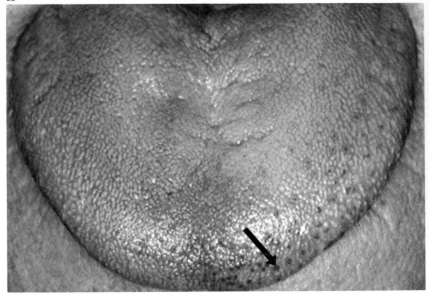

65 The taste buds These are mainly situated on the tongue and palate, and are centred on the fungiform and circumvallate papillae.

The fungiform papillae (*arrowed*) degenerate with age, and are prominent on a child's tongue. They also atrophy, as seen here on the right side of the tongue to the midline, with the loss of the chorda tympani nerve, which may be divided in ear surgery.

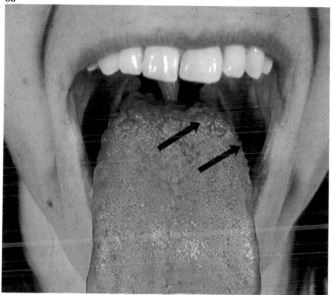

66 Circumvallate papillae These are often prominent on the base of the tongue. A patient may be alarmed when looking at the tongue to notice these normal structures and mistake them for serious disease. The foliate linguae on the margin of the tongue near the anterior pillar of the fauces may cause similar concern.

The *top arrow* indicates the circumvallate papillae. The *bottom arrow* points to the foliate linguae.

The Ear

The pinna

The pinna is formed from the coalescence of six tubercles and *developmental abnormalities* are common.

67

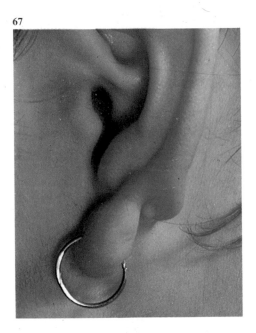

67 Minor deformities are of little importance. This shows duplication of the lobule.

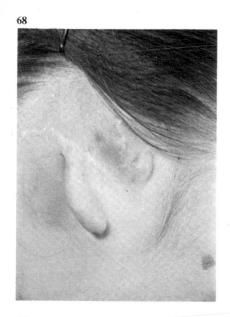

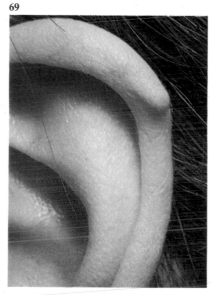

68 **Microtia** Absence of the pinna or gross deformity is often associated with meatal atresia and ossicular abnormalities. Faulty development in the 1st and 2nd branchial arches results in aural deformities
which may be associated with hypoplasia of the maxilla and mandible
and eye-lid deformities (Treacher-Collins syndrome). This type of
pinna deformity is difficult to reconstruct. Multiple surgical procedures are usually necessary and a near-normal pinna rarely
achieved. Rib cartilage grafts are taken and fashioned to act as a
scaffold for local skin rotation flaps and free skin grafts. The reconstruction is a challenge to the innovative surgeon and results vary
with the severity of pinna deformity. It may, therefore, be better to
advise no treatment or a prosthesis for gross microtia rather than
reconstruction. Prosthetics have improved greatly in recent years and
it is now possible for these to be attached to the cranium with screws
and plates (osseo-integrated implants).

69 **Darwin's tubercle** A deformity of the pinna of phylogenetic interest. It is homologous to the tip of the mammalian ear and may be
sufficiently prominent to justify surgical excision. Although Darwin's
name is used for this tubercle, Woolmer gave the first description.

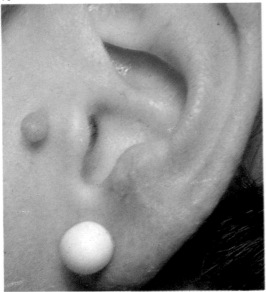

70 Hillocks (or accessory lobules) are common anterior to the tragus and are excised for cosmetic reasons. A small nodule of cartilage may be found underlying these hillocks.

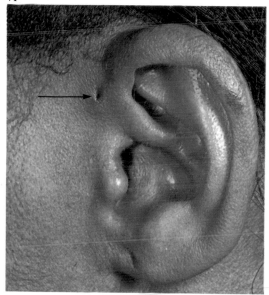

71 Pre-auricular sinuses which are closely related to the anterior crus of the helix cause more problems. Discharge with recurrent swelling and inflammation may occur, The small opening of the sinus is easily missed on examination, particularly when it is concealed, as may be the case behind the fold of the helix, rather than in the more obvious anterior site. Excision when the infection is quiescent is necessary and this, although minor surgery, is not easy. A long branched and lobular structure must be excised. If the sac is injected with a dye it is better defined. Incomplete excision of the tract leads to further infection and the need for revision surgery. Quite extensive skin loss can occur in this site with recurrent infection of a pre-auricular sinus.

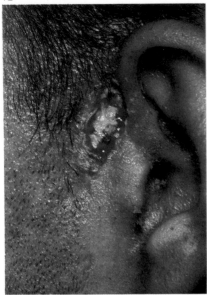 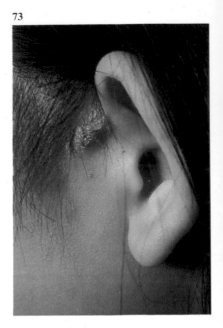

72,73 An infected pre-auricular sinus A furuncle or skin ulceration in this site is almost diagnostic of an underlying infected pre-auricular sinus.

74,75 Prominent ears The fold of the antihelix is either absent or poorly formed in a prominent ear: it is not simply that the angle between the posterior surface of the conchal cartilage and the cranium is more 'open'. Parents and child may be offended by the diagnosis of Bat or Lop ears although these terms are commonly used.

76,77 Surgical correction aims to give a natural looking ear. Modern techniques avoid a 'pinned back' appearance with a sharp tender antihelix. Reshaping of the cartilage of the pinna is necessary and recurrence follows simple excision of post-auricular skin.

Prominent ears are best corrected between the ages of four and six years at the beginning of school, but there is no additional surgical problem in correcting adult ears. Youngsters may be the subject of considerable ridicule in early years because of Bat ears and, therefore, surgical correction is not to be deferred.

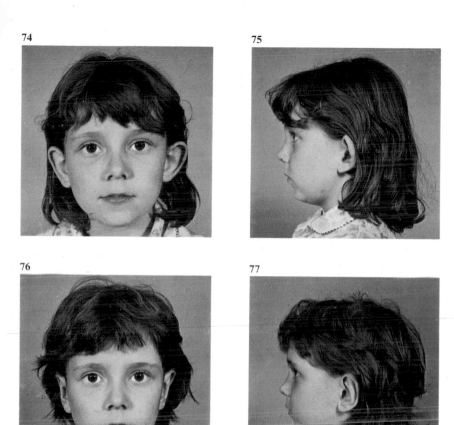

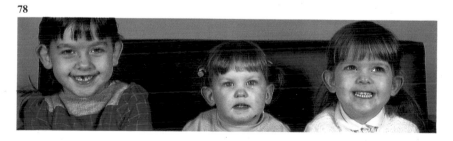

78 Bat ears are often familial and are present in all these three siblings.

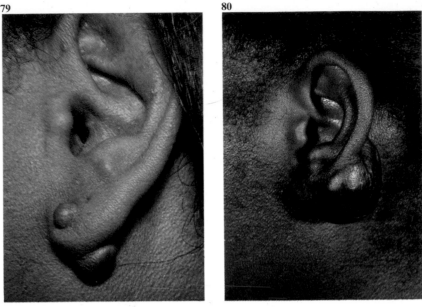

79,80 Keloid formation is common in Negroes and is difficult to treat. Recurrence follows excision and repeated excision may lead to huge keloid formation. Radiotherapy or local triamcinolone injections following excision reduce the incidence of recurrence of the keloid. Pressure at the site of keloid excision has also been shown to reduce recurrence. Special pressure clip-on ear-rings are available to apply to the ear lobe after operation. Keloid formation is common near the ear and on the neck but is almost unheard of in the middle third of the face.

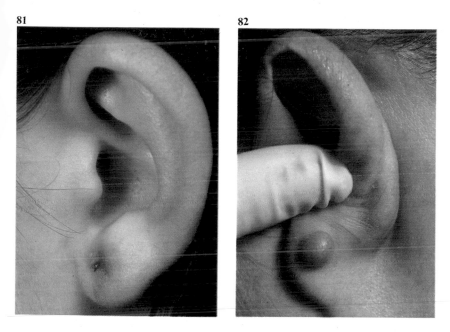

81 **Nickel sensitivity** limits the use of certain ear-rings.

82 A sebaceous cyst at the site of an ear-ring puncture. The punctum is just apparent and is diagnostic. Sebaceous cysts are common behind the ear, particularly in the post-aural sulcus.

83

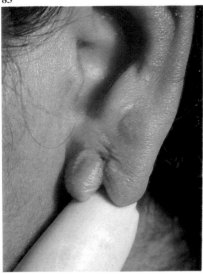

84

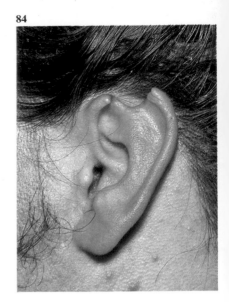

83 Traumatic 'cutting-out' when the ear-ring is pulled by a baby or adult in ill-humour. Infection at the time the sleepers are inserted is another hazard.

84 Trauma to the pinna The projecting and obvious pinna is a frequent site for trauma. Partial or complete avulsion is common; this loss of tissue is from a bite.

85 Perichondritis A painful red and swollen pinna, accompanied by fever, following trauma or surgery suggests infection of the cartilage. The organism is frequently *Pseudomonas pyocyanea*.

86 Relapsing polychondritis is a rare inflammatory condition involving destruction and replacement with fibrous tissue of body cartilage. In this case the elastic aural cartilage has been replaced by fibrous tissue so that the ear has an unusual 'felty' feel and does not have any 'spring' on palpation. The larynx too may be affected causing hoarseness which may proceed to stridor. The nasal septum may collapse. One or more of the lower limb joints are usually swollen and painful.

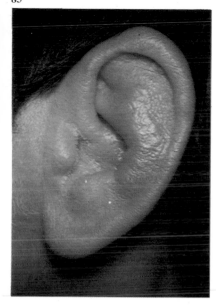

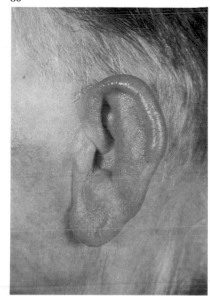

87 Collapse of the pinna cartilage followed perichondritis prior to antibiotics, and perichondritis is still a worrying complication requiring intensive antibiotic treatment. The pinna cartilage may also collapse or alter in shape in *relapsing polychondritis*.

87

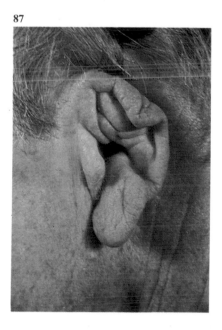

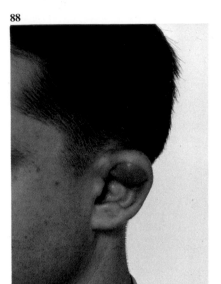 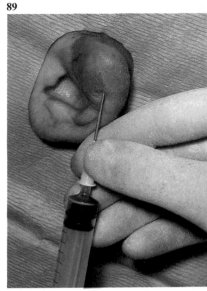

88,89 Haematomas of the pinna follow trauma. Bruising with minimal swelling settles. A haematoma or collection of serous fluid, however, is common and these, particularly, if recurrent from frequent injury and left untreated will result in a 'cauliflower ear'. The fluid if aspirated usually recurs and incision and drainage is required. Some thickening, however, of the underlying cartilage invariably takes place and a return to a completely normal-shaped pinna is not usual.

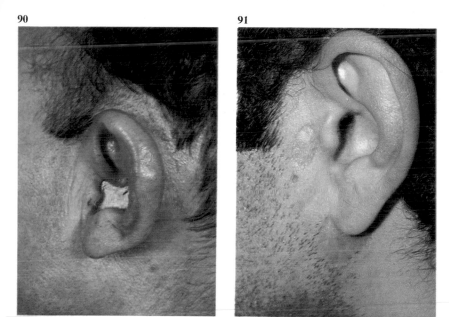

90,91 Iodoform sensitivity An antiseptic ear dressing commonly used contains bismuth, iodoform and paraffin (B.I.P.). Sensitivity to iodoform may occur and a red ear with marked irritation suggests this complication, (rather than perichondritis which is characterised by pain). Neomycin is one of the more commonly used topical antibiotics which may give rise to a skin sensitivity. Burn scars in the ear region are evidence of the past use of cautery to relieve ear symptoms in childhood. In the Arab world, these burns are still common and are known as Waxims or Chowes.

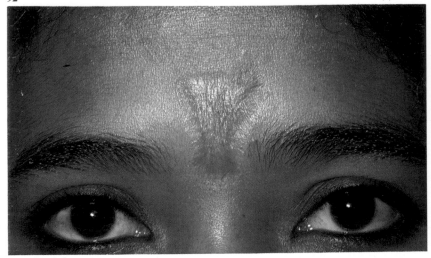

92 A Waxim in the mid-forehead where burn treatment was used in the past for headache.

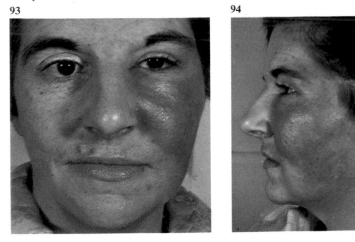

93,94 Erysipelas is caused by haemolytic streptococci entering fissures in the skin near the orifice of the ear meatus (fissures such as those in otitis externa). A well-defined raised erythema spreads to involve the face. This condition, serious in pre-antibiotic era, settles rapidly with penicillin.

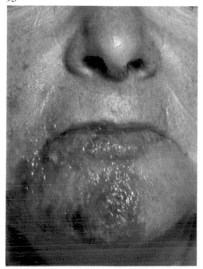

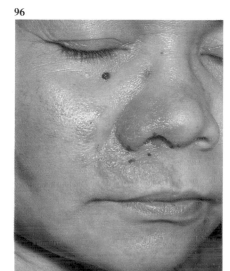

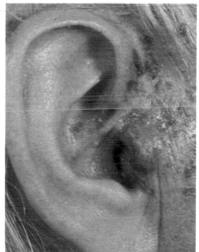

95, 96, 97 **Herpes zoster** In the head and neck, the herpes zoster virus may affect the *Gasserian ganglion* of the Vth cranial nerve. In **95** the mandibular and in **96**, the maxillary division is involved. The vesicular type of skin eruption is confined to the distribution of the nerve. The ophthalmic division of V is most frequently involved, but all three divisions of V are rarely affected at the same time.

The herpes zoster virus also involves the *geniculate ganglion* of the VIIth cranial nerve (Ramsay Hunt syndrome or geniculate herpes): herpes affects the pinna and pre-auricular region (**97**) and is associated with a facial palsy. In most cases, there is also vertigo and perceptive deafness. There is less likelihood of a full recovery of the facial palsy than in Bell's palsy.

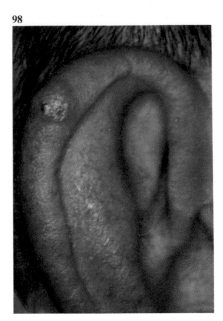 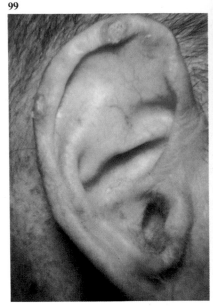

98   Basal cell carcinoma Ulceration is not uncommon on the helix; a long history suggests a *basal cell carcinoma*. This is treated with wedge resection. An ulcer of short duration suggests a squamous cell carcinoma or more rarely a melanoma, both of which require more extensive surgical resection.

99   Solar keratoses These warty growths affect the skin of the fair-headed exposed to strong sunlight. They may become malignant. The skin of the helix may be affected with several of these keratoses.

100   Inflammatory ulcers These affect the helix and occasionally the antihelix. The lesions on the helix are blessed with a lengthy diagnosis—*chondrodermatitis nodularis helicis chronicis*, which presents as a long-standing intermittent ulceration. It is primarily a chronic chondritis with secondary skin infection. A wedge resection of the ulcer and cartilage may be necessary for the ulcer does not heal with ointments.

101   Ulcers of the antihelix These are usually traumatic (on a particularly prominent antihelix fold) and are primarily a skin lesion. A basal or squamous cell carcinoma, however, may present on the antihelix.

100

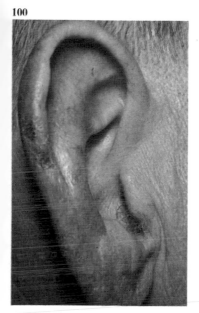

101

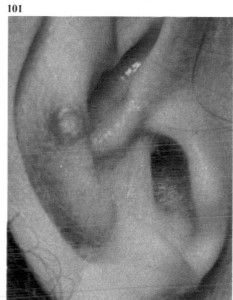

102 Gouty tophi form a characteristic lesion on the helix.

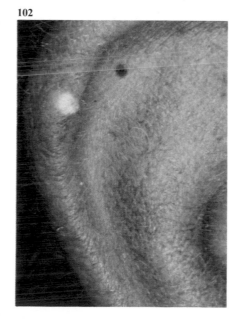

102

The external auditory meatus

The skin of the external auditory meatus is migratory and does not desquamate.

103–107 **A migrating ink dot** A dot of ink, if placed near the centre of the drum (**104**) is found to lie near the margin of the drum in 3 weeks (**105** and between 6–12 weeks the dot migrates outwards on the meatal skin (**106, 107**) to emerge in wax at the orifice of the meatus.

Cleaning of the ear canal is therefore unnecessary: those who diligently clean their ears, or those of their children, with cotton buds etc, hinder the migration of skin, and wax tends to accumulate and otitis externa develops. Some people have non-migratory skin of the external auditory meatus and are susceptible to episodes of otitis externa. The meatuses tend to become occluded with desquamated skin wax and debris and periodic cleaning of the ears is necessary. The migration of meatal epithelium is also abnormal in keratosis obturans. In this condition desquamated epithelium accumulates and may form a large impacted mass in the meatus causing erosion of the bony canal.

Skin grafts initially used for myringoplasty often failed or led to otitis externa, because skin taken from elsewhere on the body did not take on this migratory role: fascia is now used to graft the ear drum.

103

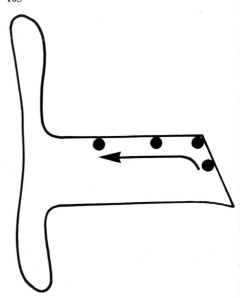

104

105

106

107

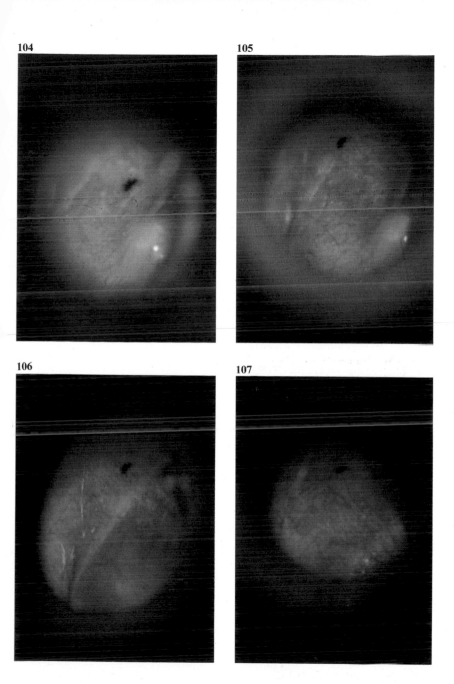

Although wax normally does not accumulate because of meatal skin migration, it may impact and cause a hearing loss.

108

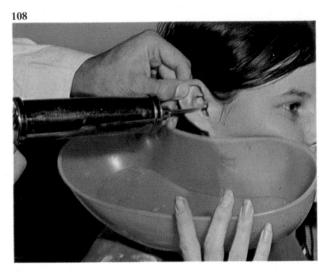

108 Syringing The rather large syringe of old-fashioned appearance has changed little in the past hundred years, and remains simple and effective treatment for wax impaction. The pinna is pulled outwards and backwards to straighten the meatus and water at body temperature is irrigated along the posterior wall of the ear. The water finds a passage past the wax, rebounds off the drum and pushes the wax outwards (**110**). Hard wax may require the use of drops before syringing.

Syringing is not painful and pain means an error in technique, or that there is an otitis externa or a perforation. If there is a perforation, an ear should not be syringed: pain with vertigo may occur with subsequent otitis media and otorrhoea; a past history of discharge suggests a perforation. Coughing (from the vagal reflex—the auricular branch of the vagus supplies the drum) or syncope may complicate syringing. Vertigo with nystagmus will occur if the water is too hot or too cold.

109

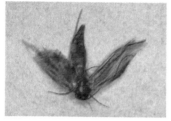

109 An insect foreign body in the ear. This insect was adherent to the tympanic membrane giving a sensation of discomfort and a deceptive drum appearance on examination: this mosquito was removed with syringing.

110

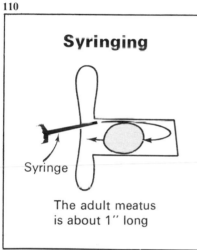

Syringing

Syringe

The adult meatus
is about 1″ long

111

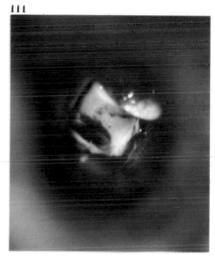

111 **Foreign body in the ear** *The main danger of a foreign body in the ear lies in its careless removal.* Syringing is very effective and safe for small metallic foreign bodies. Vegetable foreign bodies, such as peas, swell with water and are better not syringed. Insects not uncommonly become impacted in the meatus, particularly in the tropics. Maggots cause a painful ear and their removal is difficult: insufflation of pulv. calomel is usually effective treatment. Previous attempts to remove a piece of plastic wedged in the child's meatus have led to bleeding in the meatus: the drum against which the foreign body impinges can be seen deep to the plastic. One must *not* persevere in attempts to remove an aural foreign body, particularly in a child: a perforation is easily caused. If immediate removal with a hook or syringe is not effective, the patient must be admitted for removal under general anaesthetic with the help of the microscope. It is often dangerous to use forceps to remove an aural foreign body: the object easily slips from the jaws of the forceps to go deeper into the meatus.

Otitis externa Eczema of the meatus and pinna (**112**) may be associated with eczema elsewhere, particularly in the scalp, or it may be an isolated condition affecting only one ear. *Itching* is the main symptom, with scanty discharge. The eczematous type of otitis externa usually settles with cleaning of the meatus, followed by the use of a topical corticosteroid and antibiotic, but recurrence is not uncommon. The patient should avoid over-diligent cleaning of the meatus, scratching the ear, and should prevent water entering the meatus during washing or swimming: these are some of the factors predisposing to recurrence.

112

113

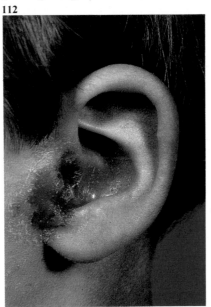 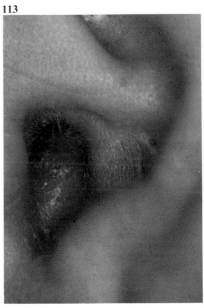

112 Ear drop sensitivity Sensitivity to ear drops may worsen an otitis externa. Chloramphenicol drops were responsible for this condition. Neomycin less commonly causes a similar reaction. Patients should be advised to discontinue ear drops that cause an increase in irritation or are painful.

113 A furuncle in the meatus is the other common type of otitis externa. It is characterised by *pain*: pain on movement of the pinna or on inserting the auriscope is diagnostic of a furuncle. Diabetes mellitus must be excluded with recurrent furuncles.

114 Furunculosis This is a generalised infection of the meatal skin. Pain is severe and the canal is narrowed or occluded so that examination with the auriscope is extremely painful and no view of the deep meatus is possible. A swab of the pus should be taken and treatment is with systemic antibiotics and a meatal dressing (eg glycerine and ichthyol, or a corticosteroid cream with an antibiotic). The organism may be transferred by the patient's finger from the nasal vestibles and a nasal swab is a relevant investigation, particularly with recurrent furuncles. The lymph nodes adjacent to the pinna are enlarged with a furuncle or furunculosis and a tender mastoid node may mimic a cortical mastoid abscess.

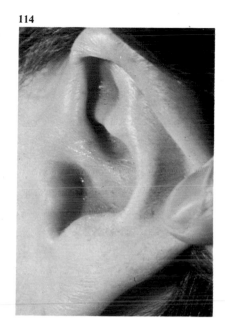

115 'Malignant' otitis externa is a rare and serious form of otitis externa to which elderly diabetics are particularly susceptible. Granulation tissue is found in the meatus infected with pseudomonas and anaerobic organisms. This granulation tissue tends to erode deeply to involve the middle and inner ear, the bone of the skull base, with extension to the brain and also the great vessels of the neck. The condition, therefore, is frequently fatal. Intense antibiotic therapy often associated with surgical drainage of the affected areas is necessary. It is not a 'malignant' condition in the histological sense for the biopsies of granulation tissue show inflammatory changes only; 'necrotising' otitis externa may be more accurate, but 'malignant' indicates the serious clinical nature.

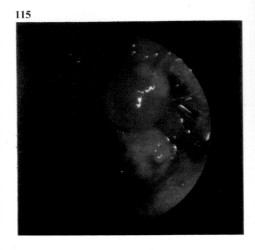

115

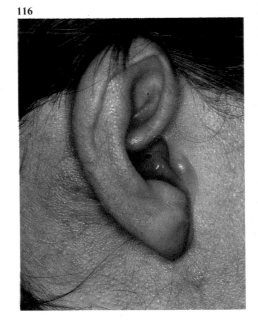

116

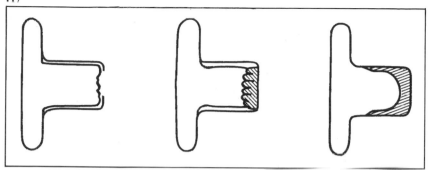

116,117,118 'Deep' otitis externa An uncommon form of otitis externa involves predominantly the skin of the deep bony meatus and the surface of the tympanic membrane. The drum epithelium may become replaced with sessile granulations infected with *Pseudomonas pyocyanea*. In protracted cases of this type of otitis externa the skin of the deep meatus and drum becomes thickened and 'funnelled' with **meatal atresia**. The resulting conductive hearing loss is extremely difficult to treat surgically once this condition is quiescent.

118

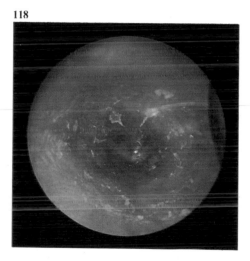

119 Otitis externa is initially treated, (an ear swab having been taken for culture and sensitivity) with cleaning of the meatus and the instillation of the appropriate antibiotic and corticosteroid drops. If the condition persists and irritation and pain are marked, a **fungal otitis externa** should be suspected. In persistent infection, the meatus contains a cocktail of drops, pus and desquamated skin. In fungal infections, as shown here, the dark spores of *Aspergillus niger* and white mycelium of *Candida albicans* can be seen. Thorough cleaning of the meatus precedes treatment with a topical antifungal agent.

The meatal skin infection is introduced from outside—usually from the patient's finger, or from water, particularly after swimming. The infection, however, may be from the middle ear if there is a perforation, and discharge from chronic otitis media may be the cause of a persistent otitis externa.

120 Bullous otitis externa (bullous myringitis) This unusual otitis externa frequently follows influenza or an upper respiratory tract infection. A complaint of earache followed by *bleeding,* followed by relief of pain is diagnostic of this condition. Examination shows haemorrhagic blebs on the drum and meatus, similar to the vesicular eruption of herpes. If there is pyrexia with a conductive hearing loss, the otitis externa is associated with an otitis media and systemic antibiotics are necessary. In the absence of pyrexia and hearing loss this condition settles spontaneously without treatment.

121 Otitis externa with herpes zoster Otitis externa occurs with herpes zoster involving either the Gasserian or geniculate ganglion, and the vesicles may be haemorrhagic. Carcinomas and melanomas in the skin of the external auditory meatus are rare but any persistent granulation should be biopsied.

119

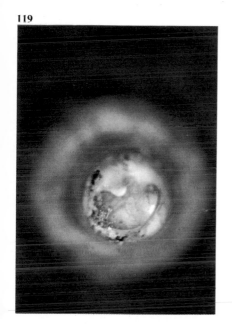

120

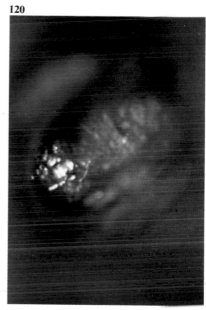

121

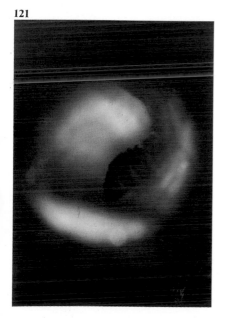

75

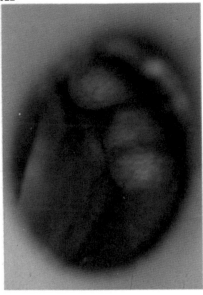
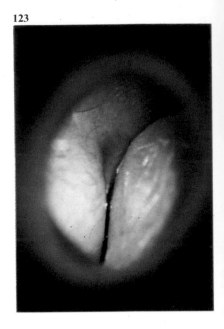

122 Osteomas White bony hard swellings in the deep meatus are a common finding during a routine examination. They usually remain small and are symptom free. They tend to be symmetrical in both ears. Swimmers are susceptible to these lesions which are sometimes called 'swimmer's osteomas'. There is experimental evidence to show that irrigation of the bony meatus with cold water produces a periostitis that leads to osteoma formation. Histologically these bony lesions are hyperostosis, rather than a bony tumour, so that the term osteoma, although established clinical diagnosis, is not strictly correct.

123 Large osteomas may narrow the meatus to a chink so that wax accumulates and is difficult to syringe. Otitis externa is also a complication. These osteomas, therefore, may require surgical removal with a microdrill. They should not be removed with a gouge, for a fracture and bleeding within the remaining osteoma is a probable complication, causing damage to the facial nerve, and resulting in facial palsy. It is rare for osteomas to occlude the meatus completely, and in almost all cases no treatment is required.

The tympanic membrane and middle ear

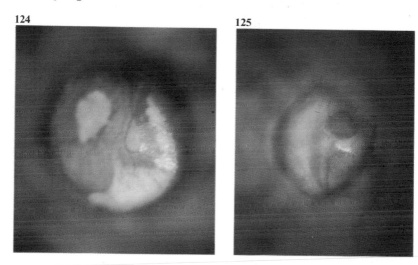

124   125

124 'Chalk' patches White areas of *tympanosclerosis* are common findings on examination of the drum. They are of little significance in themselves and the hearing is often normal. A past history of otorrhoea in childhood is usual, but chalk patches do occur with no apparent past otitis media.

Extensive tympanosclerosis with a rigid drum is a sequel of past otitis media and the ossicles, too, may be fixed or not in continuity. The chorda tympani is visible through the tympanic membrane.

125   Scarring of the drum A gossamer-thin membrane can be seen to close this previously well-defined central perforation. At first sight with the auriscope a central perforation would appear to be the diagnosis: more careful examination with a pneumatic otoscope will show that this thin membrane moves and seals the defect and reassurance that the drum is intact can be given.

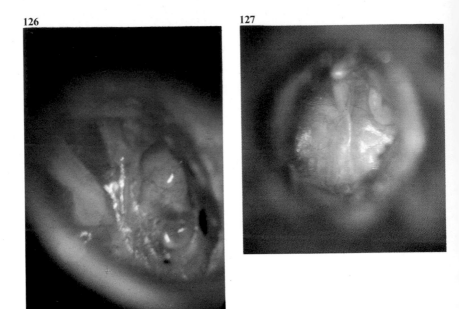

126 Scarring of the drum Scarring of the drum with retraction on to the promontory, incus and round window is also evidence of past otitis media. It is sometimes difficult to be sure whether this type of drum is intact: a thin layer of epithelium indrawn on to the middle ear structures may seal the middle ear, and examination with a Siegle's speculum or the operating microscope may be necessary to be certain of an intact drum.

127 A scarred tympanic membrane in which the drum has become atelectatic and indrawn on to the long process of the incus, promontory and round window.

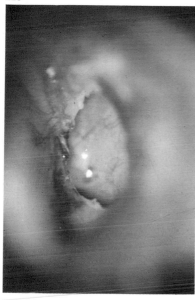

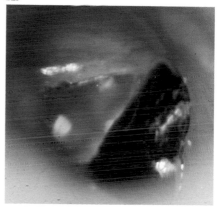

128,129,130 Traumatic perforation A blow on the ear with the hand is a common cause of a traumatic perforation which has an irregular margin and there is fresh blood or blood clot on the drum (**129**). The defect is frequently slit-shaped (**130**). Pain and transient vertigo at the time of injury are followed by a tinnitus and hearing loss.

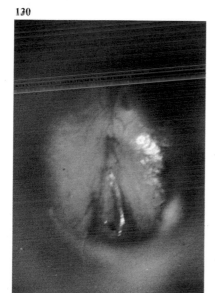

131 Healing perforation Almost all traumatic perforations heal spontaneously within two months, a thin membrane growing across the defect. Traumatic perforations are usually central but if the perforation extends to the annulus healing may not occur: the extremely large traumatic perforations also may fail to close spontaneously. Care to avoid water entering the middle ear and avoidance of inflating the middle ear with the Valsalva manoeuvre are the only precautions the patient need take. A middle ear infection with discharge is the commonest complication which usually settles with a course of topical and systemic antibiotics.

Blast injuries, barotrauma, foreign bodies or their careless removal, and even over-enthusiastic kissing of the ear may also cause traumatic perforations.

132 Central perforation Acute otitis media with pus under pressure in the middle ear may rupture the drum and although healing usually occurs, a permanent perforation can result. These perforations are usually central. A small perforation may be symptom free but episodes of otorrhoea with head colds and after swimming are common, and there is a conductive hearing loss.

The otorrhoea tends to be profuse and muco-purulent: it may be intermittent or persistent. This type of central perforation when dry is successfully closed with a fascial graft (myringoplasty). Other complications with central perforations are rare and it is described as a 'safe' perforation. A central perforation commonly persists after an episode of acute otitis media and otorrhoea in childhood; if the perforation does not close spontaneously myringoplasty is usually delayed in children for delayed closure by puberty is common. If, however, the upper respiratory tract is free of infection and the perforation is the site of recurrent infections and impaired hearing, there may be indications to proceed with myringoplasty in childhood.

133 Marginal perforation A perforation may reach the annulus posteriorly and is called marginal. The middle ear structures are frequently seen through the perforation. The well-defined margin of the round window is particularly obvious and the promontory, incudostapedial joint and stapedius are also apparent.

131

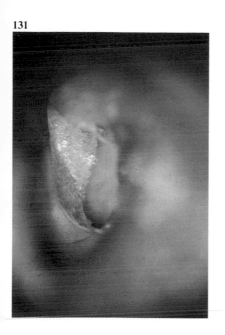

132

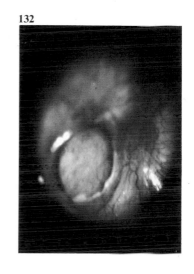

133

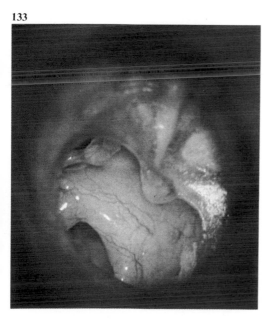

134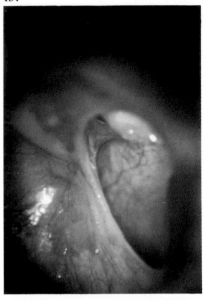

134 Squamous epithelium on the incus The marginal perforation may enable squamous epithelium to migrate into the middle ear. In this ear, white squamous epithelium has formed on the incus. Marginal perforations, therefore, are described as '*unsafe*' as there is a risk of cholesteatoma. Perforations of the pars flaccida (attic perforations) are invariably associated with cholesteatoma formation.

135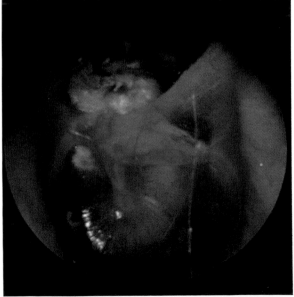

135 Attic perforation Debris adherent to the pars flaccida of the drum suggests an underlying attic perforation.

136

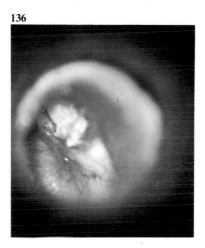

136 Cholesteatoma The debris, when removed, exposes a white mass of epithelium characteristic of a cholesteatoma. Cholesteatoma is *not* a neoplasm: it is simply squamous epithelium in the middle ear. If ignored, it increases in size, becomes infected and is associated with a scanty fetid otorrhoea. It may erode bone leading to serious complications: extension to involve the dura with intracranial infection may occur, and the facial nerve and labyrinth too may be eroded. The extent of the cholesteatoma determines the danger: a small attic pocket of epithelium is relatively harmless and can be removed with suction; an extensive mass of epithelium is dangerous and needs exploration and removal via a mastoidectomy approach. A chronic discharging ear is not painful, and persistent *pain* and headache, or severe vertigo, strongly suggest an intracranial complication or labyrinthitis.

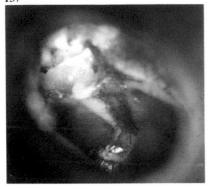
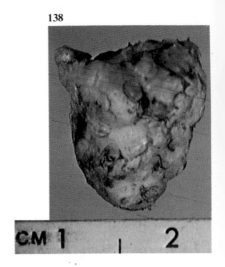

137 Cholesteatoma erodes the bony wall of the deep meatus so that a pocket containing white debris forms in the posterior-superior aspect of the drum.

The complete aetiology of cholesteatoma is not understood. Migration of epithelium into the middle ear via an attic or posterior marginal perforation certainly accounts for most cholesteatomas. Cholesteatoma, however, may occur behind an intact drum, and may form with central perforations. Eustachian tube dysfunction with a negative pressure in the middle ear, if long-standing, leads to a chronic middle ear effusion (chronic secretory otitis media) and a retracted drum. The pars flaccida retracts and may give the opportunity for a pocket of cholesteatoma to develop. In this picture of cholesteatoma, the remainder of the drum is a golden colour and fluid is present in the middle ear. The secretory otitis media may have been responsible for this cholesteatoma formation.

138 A cholesteatoma removed at mastoidectomy presents the typical well defined mass of white epithelium. The bone erosion that this mass causes shows on mastoid X-ray and particularly well on polytomograms.

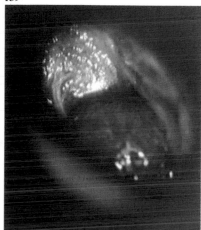

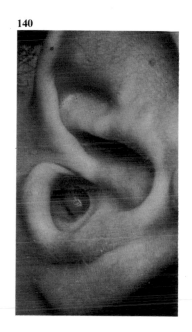

139 Aural granulation In the same way that epithelium may migrate through a perforation into the middle ear, mucous membrane may extrude outwards to the meatus. Middle ear mucous membrane extruding through a perforation becomes infected and presents with a discharging ear. An aural granulation is seen in the deep meatus. Granulation may also form on the drum at the margin of the perforation, and rarely granulation tissue forms on an intact drum in otitis externa (granular myringitis).

140 Pedunculated polyp If the growth of granulation tissue is exuberant, a pedunculated *polyp* develops, which may present at the orifice of the meatus. Granulations and polyps commonly arise from the tympanic annulus posteriorly, but the mucous membrane of the promontory, Eustachian tube orifice, and antrum and aditus may also be the site of origin.

Careful and thorough removal of polyps and granulation tissue to their site of origin is necessary. If the polyp is associated with cholesteatoma, removal by mastoid approach is required.

Mastoidectomy In the past mastoidectomy was needed for acute mastoiditis complicating acute otitis media; this was extremely common in the pre-antibiotic era and required exenteration of the mastoid air cells (cortical mastoidectomy). The operation is now rarely performed in countries where antibiotics are available.

141

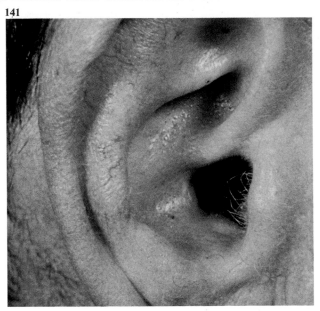

141 Enlarged meatus after mastoidectomy A more extensive type of mastoidectomy is, however, still necessary for cholesteatoma which has extended beyond the middle ear. This operation alters the anatomy of the ear. Examination after operation will show an enlarged meatus. At operation the meatus is enlarged with a meatoplasty to allow access to the mastoid cavity, so that wax can be removed with a Jobson-Horne probe or with suction. This is usually necessary once or twice a year for the skin of the mastoid cavity does not migrate satisfactorily and wax accumulates. Water entering in the ear following mastoidectomy should be avoided: infection and otorrhoea tend to follow. Syringing of a mastoid cavity is also to be avoided, not only because of the possibility of subsequent otorrhoea but irrigation of water over the exposed lateral semi-circular canal causes vertigo.

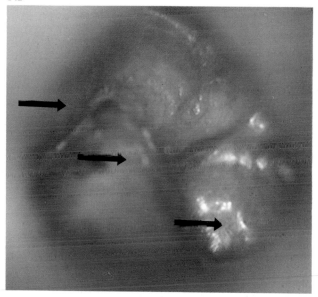

142 Auriscope view With the auriscope a ridge (which contains the facial nerve) can be seen separating the drum anteriorly from the epithelialised cavity posteriorly. Failure of the mastoid cavity to epithelialise results in an infected cavity with discharge.

Top arrow points to mastoid cavity; *second arrow* indicates the facial ridge with the bone overlying the descending portion of the facial nerve; *third arrow* shows the tympanic membrane.

Recent surgical techniques aim to remove cholesteatoma without exteriorising the mastoid cavity, so that relatively normal anatomy is maintained postoperatively, and hearing is maintained or improved (*intact canal wall tympanoplasty*), although this operation is not suitable for every case. Although avoiding a mastoid cavity, the intact canal wall tympanoplasty technique tends to conceal recurrence of cholesteatoma, and it is probable that this technique will be displaced in the future.

Secretory otitis media A sterile middle ear exudate is a common cause of conductive hearing loss. It may occur when either a head cold or barotrauma interferes with Eustachian tube function, and it often follows acute otitis media. A post-nasal space neoplasm may also cause Eustachian tube obstruction and is to be excluded in any adult with a persistent secretory otitis media.

In children secretory otitis media is very common when adenoid tissue interferes with the Eustachian tube. The middle-ear fluid **tends to be tenacious ('glue ear')**, unlike the thin straw-coloured exudate of adults.

The appearance of the drum is altered and the mobility reduced.

143

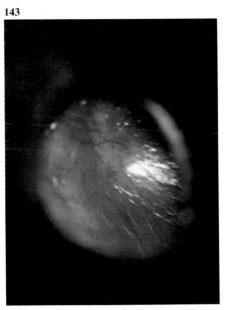

143 Secretory otitis media with minimal drum change The drum may look only slightly different with a brown colour and some hyperaemia. A confident diagnosis of middle ear fluid can only be made if reduced mobility is demonstrated and impedance audiometry (page 28) is needed for confirmation.

144

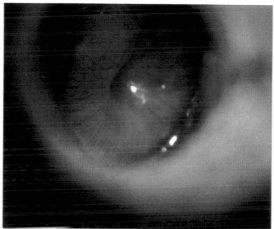

144 **Secretory otitis media (glue ear).** The *colour* change in this condition is often diagnostic, as well as the reduced mobility. The golden brown colour showing through the translucent drum is readily apparent in the inferior part of this tympanic membrane.

145

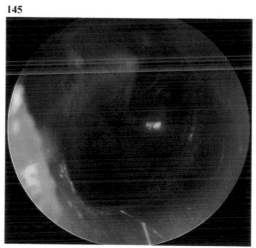

145 Secretory otitis media photographed with a fibreoptic camera giving a panoramic view of the deep meatus and membrane. Bubbles within the fluid and levels appearing as a hairline in the drum may be seen.

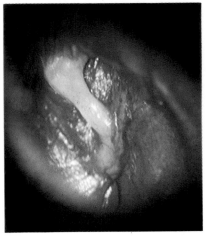 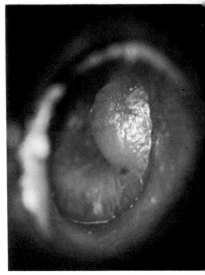

146   Secretory otitis media with marked drum change The change is frequently gross, making the diagnosis obvious, with a golden colour, a retracted membrane and a prominent malleus.

147   A vesicle on the drum also occurs in children's glue ear.

The full aetiology of the Eustachian tube dysfunction causing secretory otitis media is at present unknown. Opinions therefore differ on the treatment, particularly that of children's 'glue ears'. Adenoid tissue in the region of the Eustachian tube orifice predisposes to 'glue ears', and adenoid removal is frequently necessary surgery.

'Glue ears' are common between the ages of 3–6 years, and rarely persist after 11 years. The hearing loss is often slight and varies with colds. The self-limiting nature of the condition calls for conservative treatment, *but 'glue ears' are not to be ignored.* A marked and persistent hearing loss, interfering with schooling, necessitates surgery. Episodes of transient otalgia are common with 'glue ears', and frequent attacks of acute otitis media may occur: the drum may also become retracted and flaccid with prolonged middle ear fluid. These features may necessitate the insertion of a gromet to reventilate the middle ear. It is doubtful whether antihistamine and decongestant medicines, particularly in the absence of upper respiratory tract symptoms, have any influence on the course of 'glue ear'.

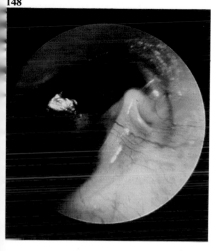 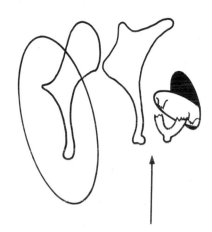

148   Blue drum The middle ear effusion evidently alters in composition, for at some stages in secretory otitis media the drum appears blue in colour—so called 'blue drum'. A similar blue appearance of the tympanic membrane is seen following injury when bleeding occurs in the middle ear (haemotympanum). The conductive hearing loss associated with this injury resolves with resorption of the middle ear haematoma. A persisting conductive hearing loss following injury, however, suggests injury to the ossicles with an ossicular discontinuity

149   Injury to the ear ossicles may follow head injury. Dislocation of the incudostapedial joint is commonest (approximately 75 per cent), but fracture of the stapes crura, and disruption of the stapes footplate also occur.

Secretory otitis media may settle spontaneously. Nasal vasoconstrictor drops with an oral decongestant (an antihistamine with a pseudoephedrine preparation) may help recovery when there is associated upper respiratory tract allergy or infection: it is doubtful, however, whether this treatment is effective in the absence of any apparent upper respiratory tract pathology. Insufflation of the Eustachian tube either by the patient performing the Valsalva manoeuvre or Politzerisation or Eustachian catheterisation may also influence recovery, but is not widely used.

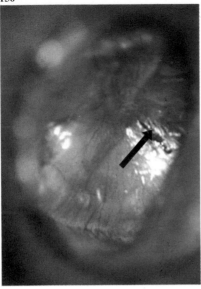

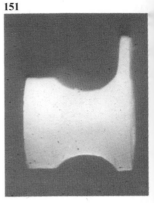

151 Gromet The insertion of a *gromet*, a flanged teflon tube, is frequently needed to avoid a recurrence of middle ear fluid.

150 Myringotomy If, however, secretory otitis media with poor hearing persists over six to eight weeks, myringotomy, usually under general anaesthetic, with aspiration of the fluid is often necessary. The arrow indicates the anterior radial incision of the myringotomy into which the gromet may be inserted.

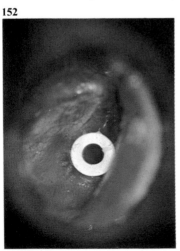

152 Gromet insertion A myringotomy incision in the posterior half of the drum may damage the incudostapedial joint or round window, and a gromet inserted posteriorly may cause incus necrosis from pressure on the long process: an anterior radial myringotomy is a safer incision for gromet insertion (as here). In both adults and children the post-nasal space must be seen to be normal.

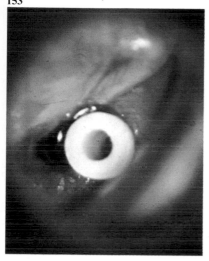

153 A gromet in place The gromet tube ventilates the middle ear and acts instead of the Eustachian tube. Hearing, and the appearance of the drum return to normal.

The gromet usually extrudes spontaneously between four to eighteen months and is found in wax in the meatus. If normal Eustachian tube function has not returned and secretory otitis media recurs, the gromet is replaced.

Obstruction of the Eustachian tube is a common and frequently diagnosed disorder. Abnormal patency of the tube, however, is also not uncommon (**the patulous Eustachian tube**) but the diagnosis is frequently missed. The condition tends to occur in people who have lost weight, women who are taking 'the pill' or are pregnant. The symptoms are of a sensation of blockage in the ear, with normal hearing or minimal loss. The patients may comment that they hear themselves breathe, eat and hear their own voice. This sensation may alter with head movement (wrongly suggesting middle ear fluid), and often is absent on lying down. Fortunately the symptoms are usually minor and settle spontaneously. Reassurance and explanation suffice as treatment in most cases. Failure to make the diagnosis, however, and treatment of the condition as Eustachian tube obstruction is common.

Chronic secretory otitis media Middle ear fluid if persistent may cause permanent changes in the drum. A secretory otitis media can cause hearing loss for decades and the diagnosis is frequently overlooked in a longstanding hearing loss. Impedance audiometry helps in diagnosis.

154

155

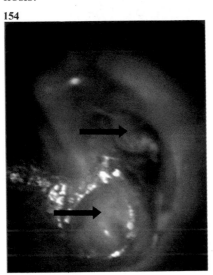 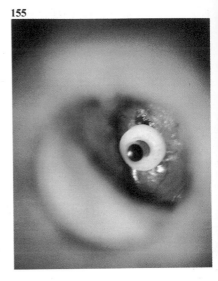

154 Grossly altered drum A brown colour, with retraction of a flaccid membrane on to the ossicles and promontory is seen. *Lower arrow* points to indrawn drum on to the promontory; *upper arrow* shows incudostapedial joint.

155 Gromet occluded with exudate Insertion of a gromet in these chronic adult cases may restore hearing but frequently the lumen of the gromet becomes occluded with exudate which may extrude through the tube into the meatus, or a constant otorrhoea occurs. There is no present successful treatment for chronic secretory otitis media failing to respond to insertion of a gromet. A further problem with chronic secretory otitis media is the return of middle ear fluid with hearing loss when the gromet extrudes. A larger flanged gromet which remains in position longer, and periodic replacement are the present remedies.

156

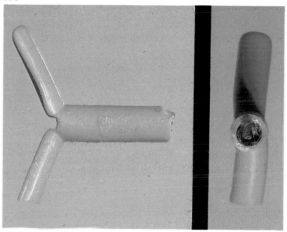

156,157   Occlusion of the gromet lumen Excess bleeding at the time of insertion may cause this problem, or subsequent occlusion with serous exudate. There are various designs of gromet or ventilation tube, and this Y-shaped tube shows the narrow lumen to be occluded.

157

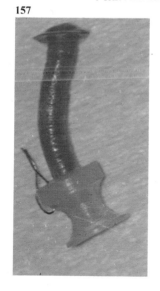

Acute otitis media Earache with conductive hearing loss and fever, accompanying a head cold, characterises acute otitis media. The drum is red and the landmarks are obscured: distension and pulsation may be seen. Otitis media is common in children, probably due to their short, wide Eustachian tube, and the presence of adenoids which may be infected near the orifice. Rupture of the tympanic membrane in acute otitis media is not uncommon and muco-purulent otorrhoea ensues with a pulsatile discharge. Penicillin is invariably curative and complications are rare. The middle ear infection frequently settles without otorrhoea but if the drum does rupture a pulsating muco-purulent discharge filling the meatus is diagnostic of otitis media. A swab for culture and sensitivity is taken in these cases although the ear usually becomes dry within 48 hours of penicillin therapy and the perforation closes in most cases with little or no scarring. Acute mastoiditis, previously serious and common, is almost unheard of where antibiotics are available. Myringotomy and cortical mastoidectomy are operations of the past for acute otitis media.

Secretory otitis media after the acute attack is the main complication today.

158

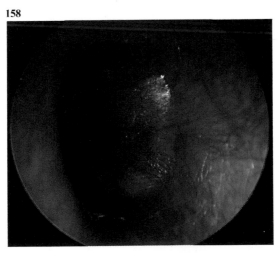

158 Acute otitis media with bulging and hyperaemia of the postero-superior quadrant of the tympanic membrane. The typical early appearance of acute otitis media photographed with a fibreoptic camera.

159

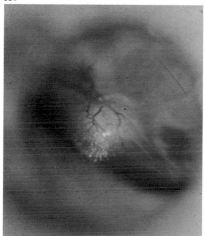

159 Glomus jugulare tumour (a chemodectoma) may present with a red drum simulating acute otitis media. *There is, however, no pain.* This tumour arises from the chemoreceptor cells near the jugular foramen and the floor of the middle ear. Pulsating tinnitus, a conductive hearing loss and a red swelling in the hypotympanum (seen here) are diagnostic of this tumour. A large tumour may extrude through the drum and present as a vascular aural polyp.

The histology is similar to the carotid body tumour, with which it may co-exist. If the glomus tumour occupies the middle ear, it can be removed via a tympanotomy or mastoidectomy approach. When the jugular foramen is involved with loss of the IX, X and XIth cranial nerves (often the XIIth from the anterior condylar foramen is also affected), the treatment is difficult. A surgical approach has been recently developed via the mastoid and neck, with a neurosurgical exposure if there is an intracranial extension. If the tumour is inaccessible surgically, radiotherapy does slow the growth of an already very slow-growing tumour and has an important place in the management, particularly in the more elderly patient. Microembolism under radiographic control of the vessels supplying the tumour is a further more modern modality used in the treatment of these very vascular lesions. If ignored, this tumour is fatal, due to intracranial spread.

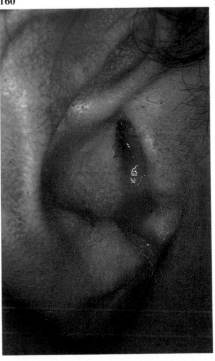

160 Bleeding from the ear, or a red or 'blue' drum (see **148, 149**) if the tympanic membrane does not rupture, may also follow base of skull fracture with bleeding into the middle ear.

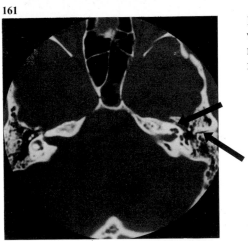

161 Base of skull fracture involving the temporal bone demonstrated on a CT scan X-ray.

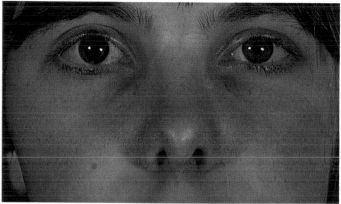

162 Otosclerosis This is a common cause of bilateral symmetrical conductive hearing loss in adults. The stapes footplate is ankylosed in the oval window by thick vascular bone: this curious bony lesion is usually an isolated middle ear focus. It may be associated, however, with osteogenesis imperfecta tarda, and *blue sclerae* are occasionally seen with otosclerosis.

Otosclerosis is familial and commoner in women (otosclerotic hearing loss increases during pregnancy and this may account for the apparent higher incidence in women). Patients frequently notice paracusis, in which they hear more clearly in noisy surroundings, unlike perceptive hearing loss in which there is difficulty in hearing with background noise. The cause of otosclerosis remains unknown.

163 The stapes The smallest bone in the body. It is, like the other ossicles, adult size at birth.

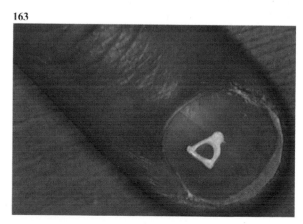

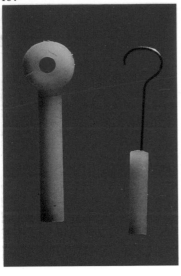

164 Stapedectomy—the prostheses
The operation for hearing loss due to otosclerosis involves removal of the ankylosed stapes bone and replacement with a mobile prosthesis. There are several types of prosthesis, of which teflon (*left*) and teflon-wire are the most commonly used. This very successful operation was devised by John Shea of Memphis, Tennessee, U.S.A., in 1957, and was a great advance in surgery with good hearing achieved in over 90 per cent of cases.

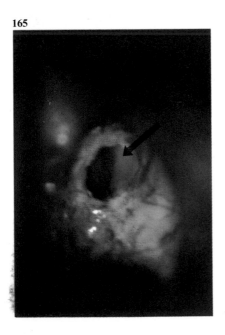

165 An opening is made in the fixed footplate (shown here). The white marks to the right of this opening into the inner ear are the otoliths.

The prosthesis is attached to the long process of the incus, and the distal end of the prosthesis is placed into the inner ear.

166

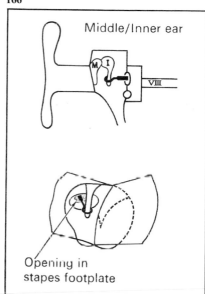

Middle/Inner ear

M I

VIII

Opening in
stapes footplate

167

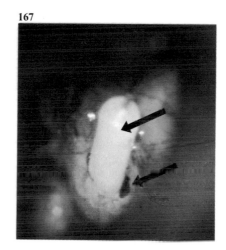

167 A teflon-wire prosthesis *(top arrow)* The distal end is entering the inner ear through the hole in the footplate *(bottom arrow)*.

166 The stapedectomy operation
The top diagram shows the attachment of the stapes prosthesis to the long process of the incus: the distal end of the prosthesis is placed through the opening made in the ankylosed stapes footplate.

The lower diagram shows the exposure of the middle ear for stapedectomy. The drum is reflected anteriorly, hinging on the long process of the malleus. The stapes superstructure and part of the footplate are removed, and the prosthesis inserted.

168

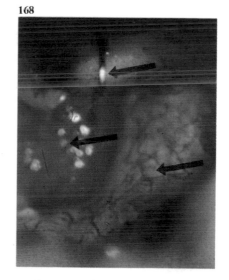

168 The wire loop is closed on to the incus *(top arrow)* and a fat graft *(second arrow)* seals the oval window. The bone covering the facial nerve *(third arrow)* and margin of the round window are also seen.

Facial palsy

169 Bell's palsy is the commonest cause of facial palsy. It is a lower motor neurone lesion of the facial nerve, of unknown aetiology, involving a loss of movement of facial muscles, usually total, of one side of the face. This includes the muscles of the forehead (with facial paralysis due to an upper motor neurone lesion, such as a stroke, these muscles continue to function due to cross innervation distal to the cortex). Pain in or around the ear frequently precedes Bell's palsy and a history of draught on the side of the face may be significant. Bell's palsy may be recurrent and associated with parotid swelling (Melkersson's syndrome). The aetiology and management of Bell's palsy is controversial. Oedema of the facial nerve near the stylomastoid foramen has been demonstrated but the cause is unknown. Most of Bell's palsies recover completely and spontaneously within six weeks. Physiotherapy maintains tone in the facial muscles during recovery, and it is probable that oral steroids (*prednisolone*) in high doses* in the early stage of Bell's improve the prognosis.

Facial palsy may follow skull fracture or facial nerve laceration near the stylo-mastoid foramen, and is also an uncommon complication of middle ear surgery and superficial parotidectomy. An extensive cholesteatoma or middle ear carcinoma may also damage the

169

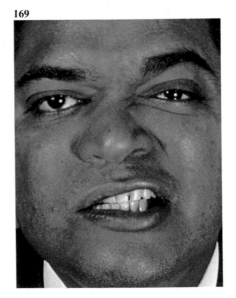

facial nerve; in the absence of a careful examination of the tympanic membrane such a case may be wrongly diagnosed and treated as Bell's palsy. All facial palsies should have an otological assessment.

Bilateral facial palsy is an interesting rarity. It is the facial asymmetry of facial palsy that is conspicuous and makes the diagnosis obvious: a bilateral facial palsy may not be so readily diagnosed.

20mgs q.d.s. 5 days: 20mgs t.d.s. 1 day: 20mgs b.d. 1 day: 20mgs o.d. 1 day: 10mgs o.d. 1 day

170,171 Tests of facial nerve involvement The level of involvement of the facial nerve in facial palsy can be determined by:

1 Taste (electrogustometry, page 47): if taste is absent or impaired the lesion is proximal to the chorda tympani.

2 Stapedial reflex (see **32** and **33**, impedance audiometry).

3 Lachrymation (Schirmer's test, **170**). Litmus paper is placed under the lower lid. If the facial nerve lesion is proximal to, or involves the geniculate ganglion, the tears are reduced.

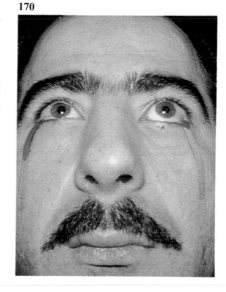

These tests are reliable in traumatic section of the facial nerve to detect the level of injury. In Bell's palsy the tests may have prognostic significance as to the successful full recovery of nerve function.

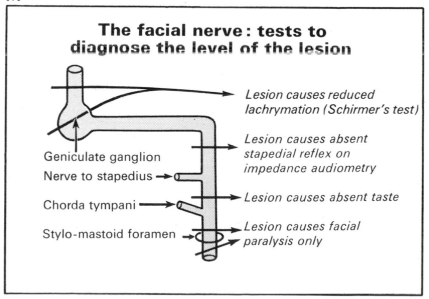

The facial nerve : tests to diagnose the level of the lesion

Geniculate ganglion
Nerve to stapedius →
Chorda tympani →
Stylo-mastoid foramen →

Lesion causes reduced lachrymation (Schirmer's test)

Lesion causes absent stapedial reflex on impedance audiometry

Lesion causes absent taste

Lesion causes facial paralysis only

Microsurgery

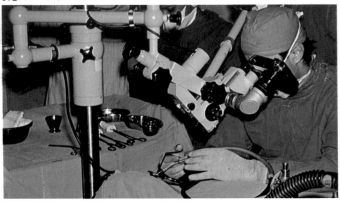

172   The middle ear operating microscope Middle ear surgery is possible because of the development of the middle ear operating microscope. This apparatus makes the drum, ossicles and other middle ear structures easy to manipulate with fine instruments.

The microscope is either sterilised with a drape or an antiseptic and a camera and tutor arm can be attached (**172**).

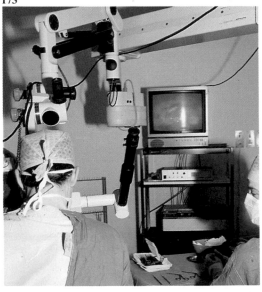

173 Operating microscope A television camera can also be attached to the microscope with a monitor giving observers a good operative view.

The Nose

Deformities

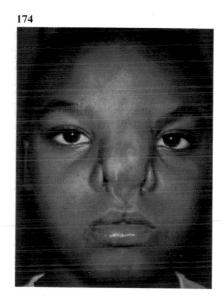

174 Congenital deformities Abnormal fusion of the nasal processes is uncommon and may result in varying degrees of deformity; in this case the nose is bifid with hypertelorism (the distance between the eyes being greatly increased). In milder cases the bifid appearance of the nose is less marked and may just appear as a rather 'wide' nose. **Congenital atresia** of one posterior choana is another congenital deformity and may not present until adult life; a total unilateral obstruction from birth may cause surprisingly little trouble to the patient. If, however, the symptoms are marked the atresia can be treated surgically with removal of the bony obstruction. Bilateral atresia presents with dyspnoea soon after birth. Immediate surgical correction is required. A membranous atresia may be perforated and dilated using metal sounds, but if the atresia is bony it must be opened with a drill using either a trans-nasal or trans-palatal approach. Indwelling portex tubes are left in place for up to 6 weeks postoperatively to prevent a recurrence of the stenosis.

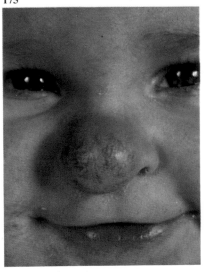

175 Haemangiomas These are seen in children and are a cosmetic problem. Treatment is deferred, for this lesion may regress before adolescence. If the deformity is gross, removal of the haemangioma with skin grafting to the defect may be necessary: cryosurgery also promises to be effective treatment, but a good cosmetic result is not easily achieved.

Cysts

176

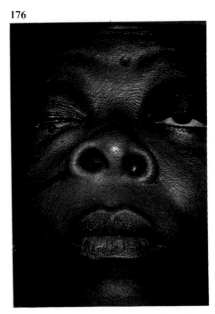

176, 177 Naso-alveolar cysts This is more common in Negroes and its constant anatomical site makes spot diagnosis possible. Externally there is flattening of the naso-labial fold and flaring of the alae nasi. In the anterior nares the cyst extends into the floor of the nose and displaces the inferior turbinate upwards. Excision via a sublabial incision and enucleation is the treatment. Surgical rupture of the cyst usually means incomplete removal and predisposes to recurrence. *Arrow* indicates 'flaring' of ala.

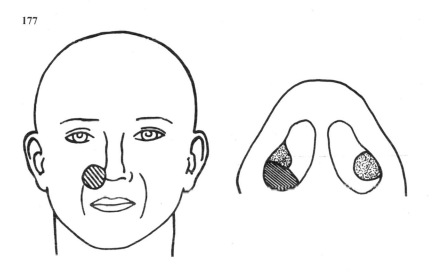

178 **Dermoid** A cystic swelling near the glabella is probably a dermoid; excision is straightforward The differential diagnosis in childhood is the *nasal glioma*. This unusual nasal tumour is benign and presents either externally or as an intranasal swelling. It is either a completely separate firm tumour, or is connected to the cerebrum through a dehiscence in the cribriform plate. X-rays to exclude an intracranial origin are necessary before a nasal glioma is excised.

178

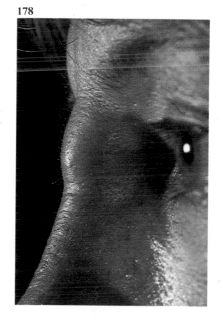

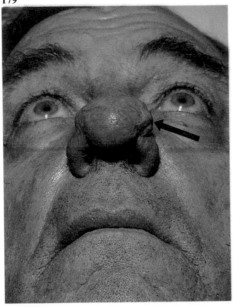

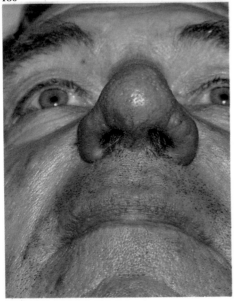

179, 180 Rhinophyma is the nasal deformity from advanced acne rosacea in which the skin epithelium becomes grossly thickened and vascular. 'Shaving' of the excess skin (without skin grafting) is the surgical treatment. Irregular areas of epithelium (*arrow*) should be sent for histology, for basal or squamous cell carcinoma may occur within a rhinophyma.

Adenoids

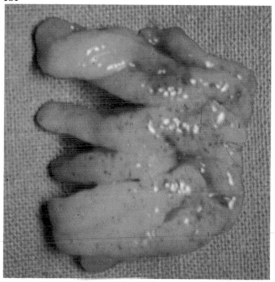

181 Adenoids A mass of lymphoid tissue shaped like a bunch of bananas, occupies the vault of the post-nasal space in children. If the adenoids are large, nasal obstruction occurs. There is snoring, with purulent rhinorrhoea if there is a secondary sinusitis, and epistaxis. Aural symptoms due to interference with the Eustachian tube also occur, with or without nasal symptoms; there is hearing loss due to secretory otitis media, or earache from recurrent acute otitis media.

Adenoids normally regress before puberty and adults with large adenoids are rare. If an adult has nasal obstruction due to post-nasal lymphoid tissue, the histology is essential to exclude a lymphosarcoma. Nasal obstruction may occur from birth due to large adenoids, and the baby has difficulty with bottle and breast feeding. It is occasionally necessary to remove these 'congenital adenoids' in toddlers. A conservative attitude should be taken, however, with removal of adenoids, awaiting natural regression of the lymphoid tissue; only marked nasal and aural symptoms necessitate operation.

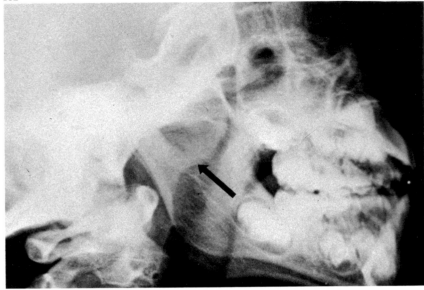

182   Lateral X-ray of adenoids The post-nasal space is often difficult or impossible to see in a child and a lateral X-ray shows clearly the size of the adenoids and degree of obstruction. In this X-ray a small airway is present despite a large adenoid shadow.

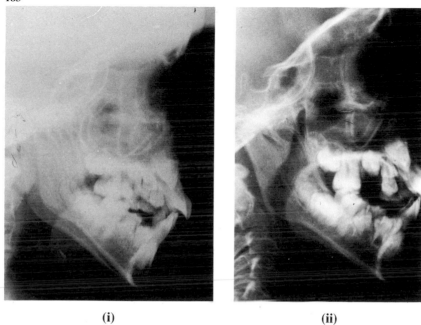

(i)   (ii)

183 It is necessary to have an accurate lateral X-ray A wrongly angled X-ray demonstrated here (**i**) is not infrequently erroneously reported as showing 'large adenoids'. It is not easy to maintain a child in the correct position. Patience and skill are required by the Radiographer. When checking the lateral X-ray for adenoids, therefore, it is essential to be sure that the lateral picture is true (**ii**) before assessing the bulk of adenoid lymphoid tissue.

Trauma

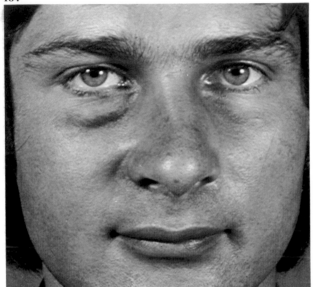

184 Fractured nose This common injury only requires treatment if the septum is dislocated or involved in haematoma, or if there is an external deviation of the nose (seen here and most obvious when examined from above **185**) of cosmetic concern to the patient. It is important to reduce nasal fractures within two weeks, lest the bones cannot be manipulated and a subsequent rhinoplasty or re-fracture may be necessary. Reduction, therefore, is carried out either soon after fracture or is delayed until the oedema, which makes assessment of the deformity difficult, has settled.

Many fractured noses, however, are 'chip' or undisplaced crack fractures with haematoma, and require no treatment.

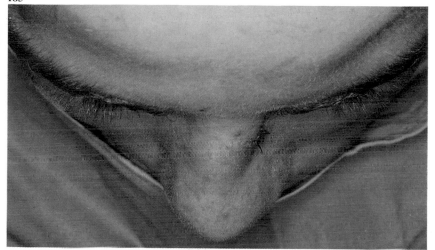

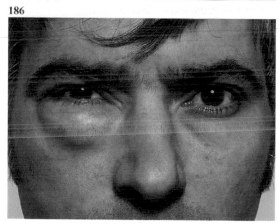

186 An alarming and unusual complication of a nasal fracture is surgical emphysema of the orbit when the patient blows the nose. This is due to a fracture through the ethmoidal cells and lamina papyracea linking the nasal cavity to the orbit. There is no cause for alarm, and care not to inflate the orbit is followed by spontaneous healing. The characteristic crepitus on palpation is diagnostic. A facial injury that has caused a nasal fracture may also have involved the maxilla and anterior cranial fossa (with C.S.F. rhinorrhoea) and precautions should be taken to exclude such an associated fracture as well as any possible injury to the eye.

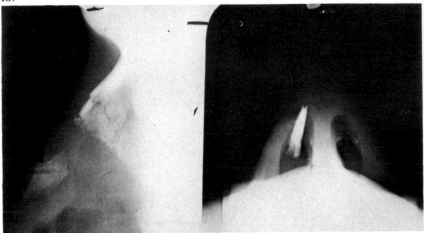

187 X-ray of nasal bones showing complete separation of one bone. In this case the nasal bone X-ray shows some obvious and significant injury. In almost all instances, however, the X-rays for a fractured nose are of very little practical value, although they may be of medico-legal significance.

Complications of a fractured nose

One complication of a fractured nose is a **septal haematoma**. If this causes *complete* nasal obstruction surgical drainage is necessary. If the nasal obstruction is partial, it is probable that the haematoma will settle spontaneously without treatment. Secondary infection may occur and is characterised by pain. Incision of the septum and drainage is necessary. The patient must be warned *before* operation that a **saddle deformity** (as here) due to lack of septal support may develop following a haematoma. A septal haematoma may also follow surgical correction of a deviated septum (submucous resection).

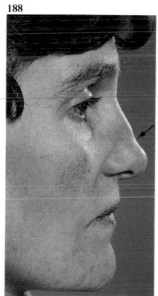 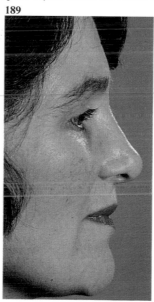

188 **Minimal saddling,** as in this patient, may accentuate a previous nasal hump. Simple lowering of the nasal bones restores the appearance of a normal nose (**189**).

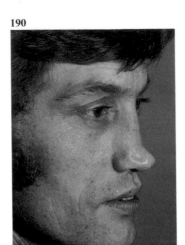
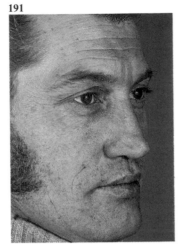

192

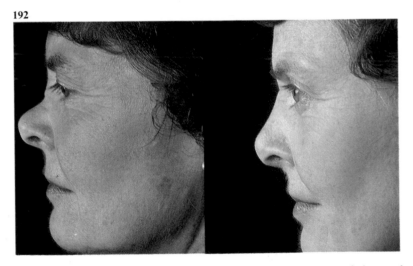

190-192 With the more common severe saddling, a graft is needed to restore the nasal contour. Cartilage, bone, or a synthetic are alternative grafting materials.

193

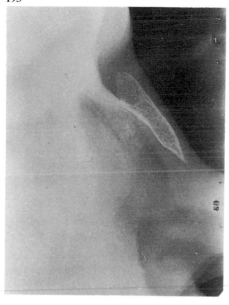

193 An iliac crest bone graft used for a saddle deformity is demonstrable on this X-ray.

194

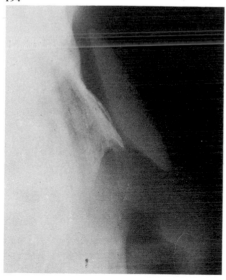

194 A synthetic graft (silastic) seen on X-ray, is also used to correct nasal saddling.

195

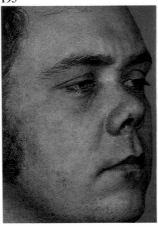

196

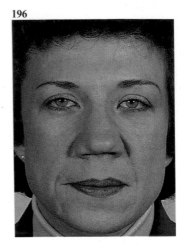

195 Septal haematomas are not uncommon in children and may be spontaneous, in which case a blood dyscrasia needs to be excluded, or follow trauma. The parents should be warned that the development of the nose may be retarded and ultimately lead to a 'small' nose in adult life. In the past surgical correction was left until the nose was fully grown at the age of 16-17 years, but it is now apparent that grafting of these saddle deformities in childhood will lead to more normal nasal development.

196 Retraction of the columella and loss of tip support of the nose are less usual complications of a septal haematoma.

197-200 Nasal saddling following trauma at the age of seven years, and the development of a normal adult nose with grafting.

197

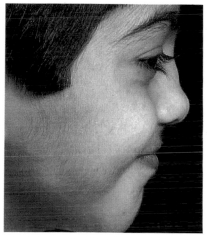
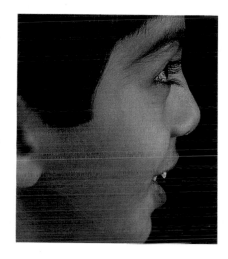

Before grafting   **After grafting**

198

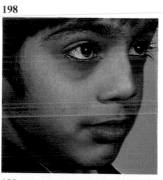

197 Aged 7 years

198 Aged 11 years

199 Aged 15 years

200 Aged 19 years

199

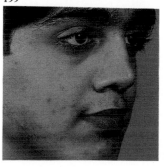

200

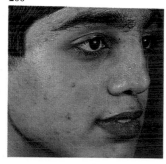

Rhinoplasty The appearance of a nose with a congenital or traumatic hump of the nasal bones can be improved with rhinoplasty (**201-203**). A deviated nose may be straightened (**204,205**). Bulbous or bifid nasal tips can be modified (**206**). Incisions for rhinoplasty are within the nasal vestibule and access to the nasal bones, cartilages, and septum is obtained with an intranasal approach.

201

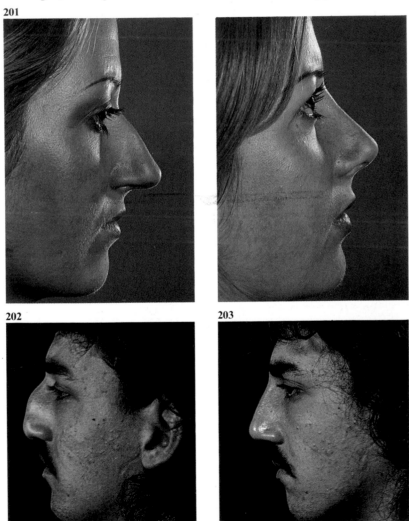

202

203

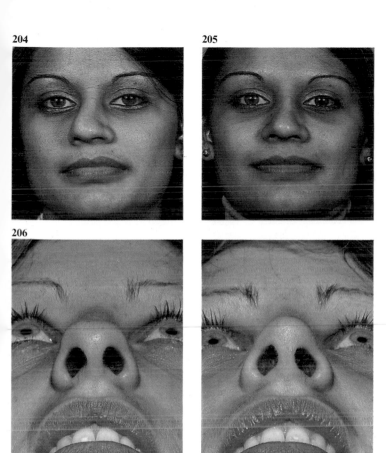

Mentoplasty The improvement with rhinoplasty in this case has been accentuated by mentoplasty (**207-209**). A silastic implant has been inserted adjacent to the mandible (**209**). A receding chin is not to be overlooked in a patient seeking rhinoplasty, for it accentuates the nasal deformity, and mentoplasty gives a subtle but striking appearance improvement.

207
208

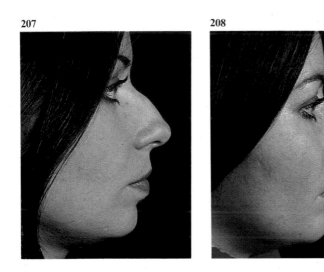

209

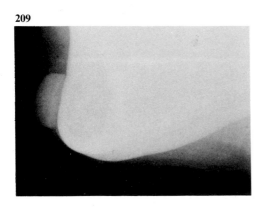

Deviated nasal septum A congenital or traumatic dislocation of the septal cartilage into one nasal fossa causes unilateral nasal obstruction. If the obstruction is marked, or complicated by recurrent sinusitis, a septal correction is minor and effective surgery. The established and time-honoured operation for this is the submucous resection (SMR) but septoplasty techniques in which cartilage is preserved and repositioned—rather than removed—are now more widely used. The SMR operation involves removal of much of the septal cartilage and loss of nasal support with saddling, and septal perforations are occasional complications.

210

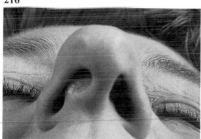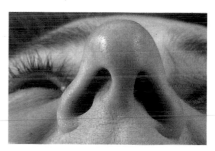

210 Deviated nasal septum into the columella With caudal dislocation of the septum, an obvious deformity is coupled with nasal obstruction. Repositioning or excision of the septal dislocation is necessary to improve the appearance and airway.

211 Deviated nasal septum with a spur of septal cartilage and maxillary bone occluding the inferior meatus and causing *nasal obstruction*.

211

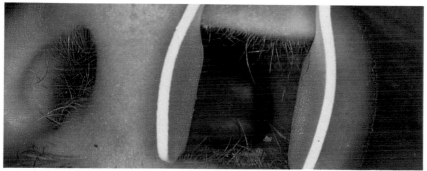

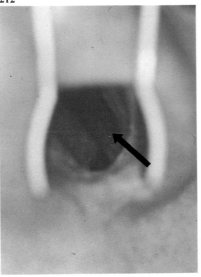

212 Septal spur indenting the inferior turbinate A posterior deviation of the septum can be overlooked, and a vasoconstrictor applied to the anterior nasal mucous membrane reduces the size of the turbinates and allows a clear view posteriorly. *Arrow* indicates septal spur.

213

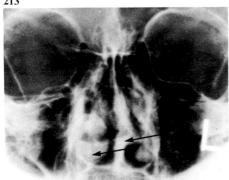

213 A posterior septal deviation Such deviations of the vomer and ethmoid bone show on X-ray (*upper arrow*). Also seen on X-ray is the *compensatory hypertrophy of the inferior turbinate* on the opposite side to the deviation (*lower arrow*). It is necessary to reduce this turbinate when the septum is straightened, lest this nasal fossa becomes obstructed postoperatively.

214 Deviated nasal septum in a child The diagnosis is obvious without the use of a nasal speculum. Elevation of the infantile nasal tip suffices to give a clear view of the anterior nares.

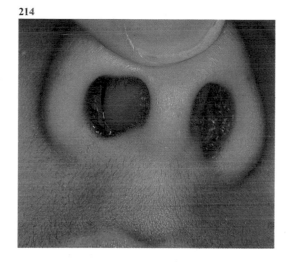

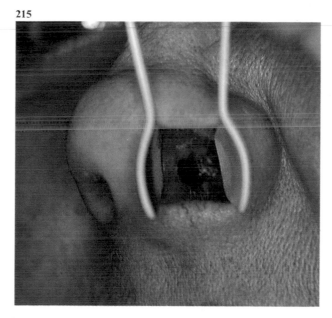

215 A perforation of the nasal septum This may give rise to no symptoms and be a chance finding on examination. Crusting usually occurs, however, and causes nasal obstruction.

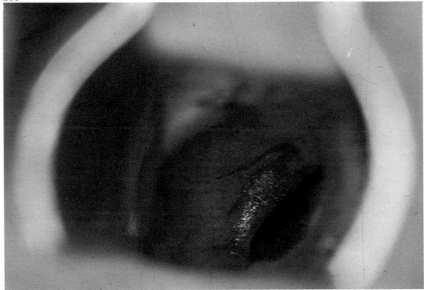

216 Prominent blood vessels appearing on the margin of the perforation: these lead to epistaxis. A whistling noise on breathing is another symptom.

Perforations may result from repeated trauma to the septum (eg nose picking); chrome workers are susceptible to a septal perichondritis causing a perforation. An inadvertent tear of the nasal mucous membrane on both sides during an SMR operation is another cause of perforation. Destruction of the vomer and ethmoid bone accounts for a posterior septal perforation, and may be due to a gumma. Surgical repair of septal perforations, particularly large ones, is not easy. Composite cartilage grafts taken from the concha of the ear combined with mucosal rotation flaps of the nasal mucous membrane form the basis of most current techniques. Plastic flanged prostheses may be fitted to seal the perforation but may extrude and also be inhaled.

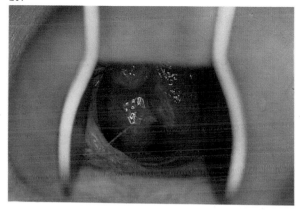

217 Granulation tissue in the nose requires biopsy. **Sarcoidosis** not infrequently involves the upper respiratory tract mucosa of the nasal fossae and larynx. In the nose the granulations are pale, but tuberculosis, malignant granuloma and neoplasia are among the differential diagnoses.

218

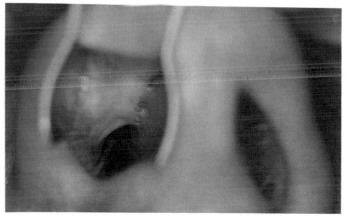

218 Nasal adhesion Adhesions or synechiae may follow nasal trauma (including surgical trauma) and bridge the lateral wall of the nose, frequently from the inferior turbinate to the septum, causing nasal obstruction. Recurrence follows surgical division of the larger adhesions unless an indwelling silastic splint is left *in situ* until mucosa underlying the adhesion regenerates.

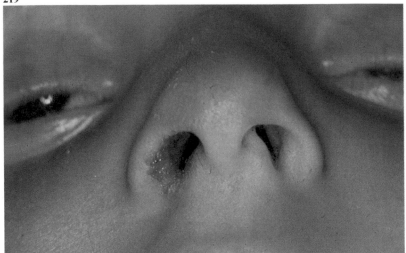

219 A foreign body in the nose causes a unilateral purulent and fetid nasal discharge. A child with these symptoms and a vestibulitis is almost certain to have a foreign body in the nose.

220

220 Vestibulitis affecting one nostril, as in this case, is almost always diagnostic of a foreign body.

221 When nasal discharge and skin involvement affect both nostrils, a vestibulitis (an eczema of the vestibular skin) is the probable diagnosis.

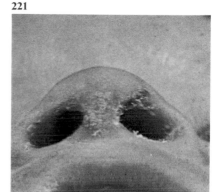

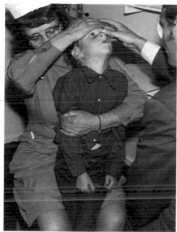

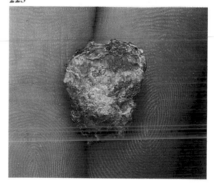

222   Removal of a foreign body Removal frequently can be managed as an outpatient, when it is necessary to hold the child securely while a probe or hook is placed posterior to the foreign body: forceps frequently push the foreign body posteriorly and should be avoided. A general anaesthetic is necessary if the foreign body is impacted or inaccessible.

223   A foreign body that is ignored accumulates a calcareous deposit and presents years later as a fetid stony hard mass—a **rhinolith**. This is well demonstrated on X-ray and a rhinolith may become large eroding the lateral wall and floor of the nose. Although at first sight appearing easy to remove, the impaction may be extremely firm particularly with the larger rhinoliths.

Inflammation

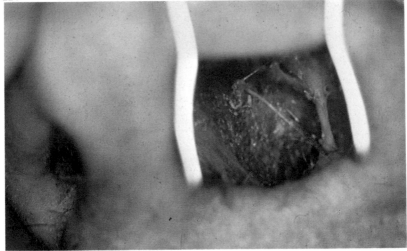

224 **Vestibulitis** presents as crusting and irritation in the anterior nares with nasal obstruction. Examination shows excoriated vestibular skin and septal mucous membrane. Rubbing or over-diligent cleaning of the nose by the patient usually causes vestibulitis particularly if, as in this case, the septum is deviated anteriorly and impinges on the lateral wall of the nose. Advice and the use of antibiotic and corticosteroid ointment control vestibulitis. Correction of the septum may be necessary.

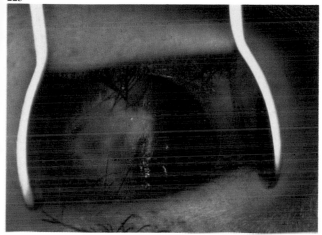

225 Nasal vestibulitis with squamous epithelium replacing the mucosa A deviation of the septum has predisposed to a chronic vestibulitis. Digital irritation, or the **use of cocaine** which may also lead on to a septal perforation may underlie this problem. Despite the increased use of cocaine gross septal damage in cocaine sniffers is not very common.

226

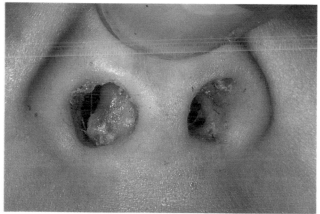

226 Vestibulitis in a child overlying a grossly deviated anterior septum Septal surgery is avoided in children but cases in which the obstruction is gross with vestibulitis require a conservative septoplasty.

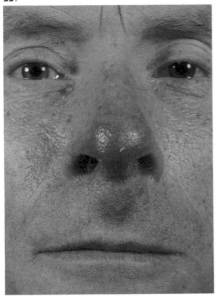

227, 228 Furuncles and cellulitis of the columella These may spread to involve the skin of the nose and face. Treatment is with systemic penicillin.

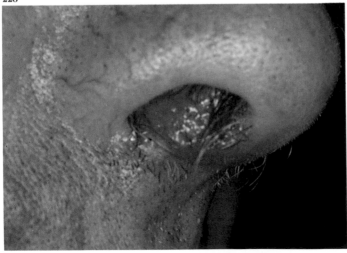

229

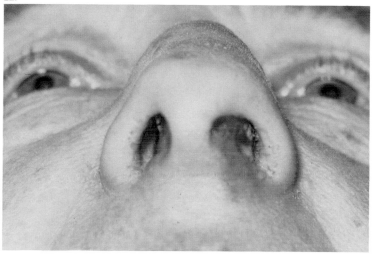

229 Vestibulitis Painful crusting of the nasal vestibule and anterior nares may be a simple eczematous type of skin lesion which settles with a topical antibiotic and steroid. There should be, however, an awareness that this vestibulitis is a granuloma, or part of the manifestation of systemic disease such as polyarteritis nodosa or systemic lupus erythematosus. A further possibility is an 'irritative' vestibulitis from cocaine snuff, or columellar carcinoma, as in this case.

230

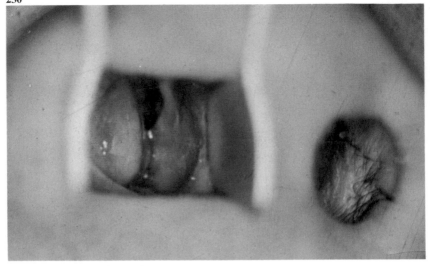

231

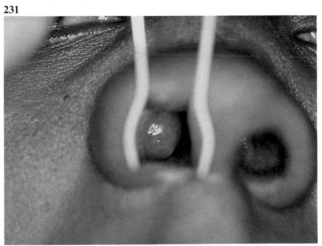

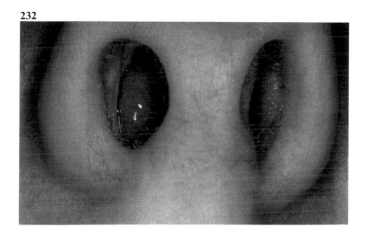

230-232   Acute rhinitis In the common cold the nasal mucous membrane is oedematous, so the inferior turbinate abuts against the septum causing obstruction, and there is an excess of mucus causing the running nose. A similar appearance is seen in *nasal allergy*, either 'seasonal hay fever', or perennial allergy, but the oedematous turbinate mucous membrane appears grey (**232**) rather than red (**231**). A persistent purulent nasal discharge usually means that there is a sinusitis. Specific nasal sprays for nasal allergy are now available markedly reducing the obstruction, rhinorrhoea and sneezing that characterises both seasonal and perennial nasal allergy. Skin tests to detect specific allergens are of use with grass pollen and house dust allergy related to the house dust mite. Nasal sprays (such as Beconase), desensitisation and the oral antihistamines are the main lines for treatment of nasal allergy. Antihistamines without sedative side-effects have become available more recently. This management of nasal allergy is preferred to desensitisation for which good results are not well proven and there is an increased awareness and concern regarding anaphylactic shock.

233

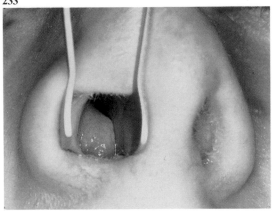

233 Chronic rhinitis The turbinate mucous membrane frequently reacts to irritants whether tobacco, excessive use of vasoconstrictor drops or atmospheric irritants, by enlarging. Thickened red inferior turbinates are seen adjacent to the septum limiting the airway (**233**). Nasal obstruction either intermittent or persistent, with a post-nasal discharge of mucus (post-nasal 'drip') are the symptoms of chronic rhinitis. This is the condition most frequently labelled by the patient as 'catarrh' or 'sinus trouble'. If the changes due to the chronic rhinitis are irreversible, ie the nasal obstruction persists when the irritants are removed, it is probable that minor surgery to reduce the turbinates in size will be necessary. Occasionally, oral antihistamines help, but vasoconstrictor drops have no place in the treatment of chronic rhinitis and their constant use is a common cause of this condition (*rhinitis medicamentosa*).

In most inflammatory conditions of the nasal mucous membrane there is an excess of mucus. An atrophy of the mucosa and mucous glands with fetid crusting of wide nasal fossae, however, is seen with *atrophic rhinitis*. This is uncommon and idiopathic: it may be an isolated nasal condition or part of Wegener's granuloma or disseminated lupus erythematosus. There is also a phase of atrophic nasal crusting in rhinoscleroma.

234,235 Acute maxillary sinusitis This is a common complication of a head cold. Apical infection of the teeth related to the antrum, or an oro-antral fistula following dental extraction also cause maxillary sinusitis, as may trauma with bleeding into the antrum, or barotrauma. Frontal or facial pain may be referred to the upper teeth.

Nasal obstruction and purulent rhinorrhoea are the other symptoms. The antrum is *opaque* on X-ray (**235**) and dull on transillumination. There may be tenderness over the sinus but swelling is rare. Pus is seen issuing from the middle meatus (**234**).

Acute infection may less commonly affect the ethmoid, frontal and sphenoid sinuses. Systemic antibiotics, a vasoconstrictor spray or drops, and inhalations are usually curative for acute sinusitis. A persistent maxillary sinusitis, however, requires an antral washout.

234

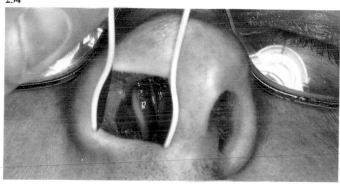

235

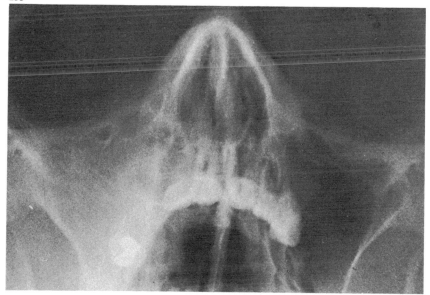

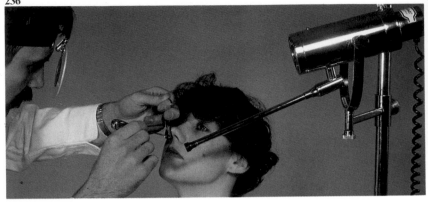

236,237 An antral washout This involves inserting a trocar and cannula under the inferior turbinate, and puncturing the lateral wall of the nose through the maxillary process of the thin inferior turbinate bone, to enter the antrum. Water is irrigated through the cannula and the pus emerges through the maxillary ostium. *An acutely infected maxillary sinus must **not** be washed out, until medical treatment has controlled the acute phase; cavernous sinus thrombosis remains a danger.* The bad reputation that antral washout has for pain is not justified if a good local anaesthetic and gentle technique are used.

Recurrent attacks of acute maxillary sinusitis may require operation.

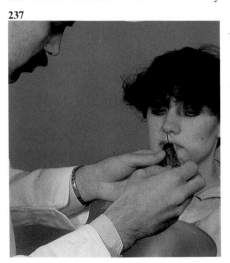

237

A permanent intranasal opening into the antrum is made either in the middle or inferior meatus (**intranasal antrostomy**). This operation is also effective for those cases of acute sinusitis that fail to respond to conservative treatment and antral washouts.

238 Dental sinusitis The apices of the molar teeth may be extremely close to the antral mucosal lining. The upper wisdom tooth apparent on this X-ray, if infected, would be likely to cause maxillary sinusitis or, if removed, would be clearly at risk to cause an oro-antral fistula.

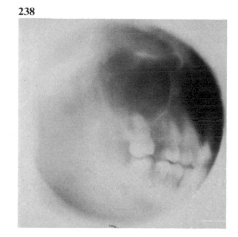

238

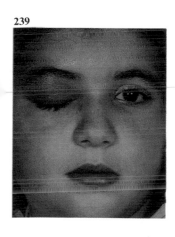

239

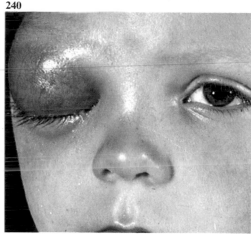

240

239 Orbital cellulitis Complications of acute sinusitis confined to the antrum are rare. A severe maxillary sinusitis, however, usually involves the ethmoid and frontal sinuses. Infection spreading via the lamina papyracea or floor of the frontal sinus leads to an *orbital cellulitis*.

240 Orbital abscess requiring external drainage may form. Meningitis or brain abscess may also follow spread of infection from the roof of the ethmoid, frontal or sphenoid sinus to the anterior cranial fossa. Infection associated with a rapidly growing neoplasm, such as a **rhabdomyosarcoma**, is the differential diagnosis in this case.

Chronic sinusitis This may develop from incomplete resolution of an acute infection. The onset, however, may be insidious and secondary to nasal obstruction (eg due to a deviated septum, nasal polyps or, in children, to enlarged adenoids). Apical infection of the teeth related to the antra can also cause chronic sinusitis.

Purulent rhinorrhoea, nasal obstruction and headache are the main symptoms of chronic sinusitis. Pus in the middle meatus with opacity of the sinus are confirmatory of infection. Pus confined to the antrum rarely gives complications, but often there is spread of infection to the ethmoids and frontal sinuses. It is not common for frontal and ethmoidal sinusitis to occur without maxillary sinusitis. Pus in the frontal and ethmoid sinus, as with acute infections, may spread to involve the orbit and brain. Obstruction of the sinus ostium may lead to an encysted collection of mucus within the sinus—a mucocele.

241

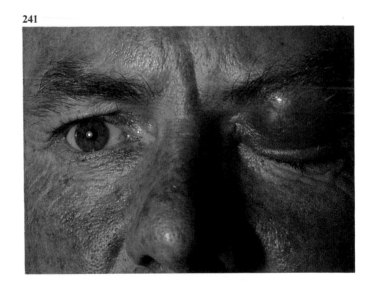

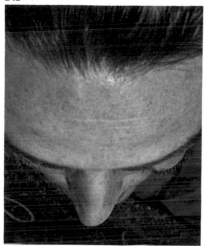

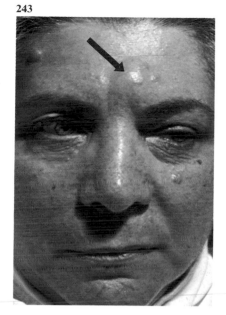

241-243 A mucocele The frontal sinus is commonly affected and erosion of the roof of the orbit leads to orbital displacement downwards and laterally. Proptosis also occurs and is best confirmed by examination from above (**242**). The frontal sinus wall may be eroded both posteriorly and anteriorly. An eroded anterior wall results in a fluctuant swelling on the forehead (**243**). In this case there is also orbital displacement and proptosis.

244

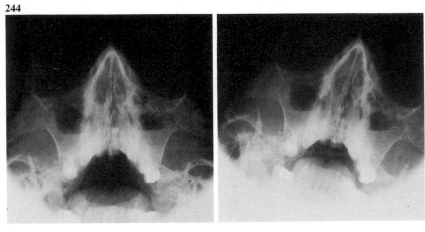

245

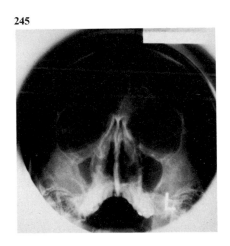

246

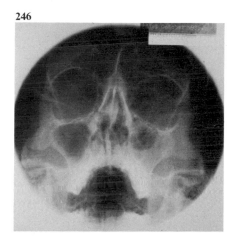

247

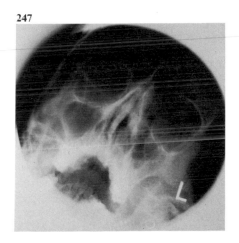

244-247 Maxillary sinus X-rays In acute and chronic maxillary sinusitis fluid may be seen on X-ray. It is essential if a *fluid level* is seen for a tilted view to be taken to confirm the presence of fluid (**244**). A thickened (**245**), or rather 'straight' mucous membrane (**246**) may look like a fluid level, as may a bony shadow if the X-ray is wrongly angled. Tilting confirms fluid (**247**).

248 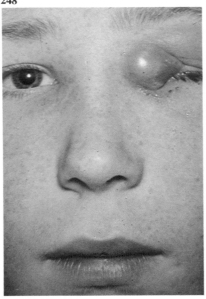 **249**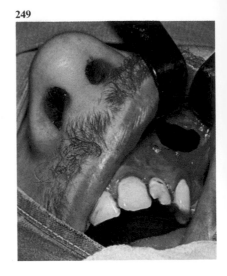

248 Lateral displacement of the orbit This occurs with a mucocele arising in the ethmoid sinus and is usually accompanied by swelling at the medial canthus. In this case the mucocele is infected—*a pyocele*.

249 The Caldwell-Luc operation Chronic maxillary sinusitis may require the Caldwell-Luc operation in which the antrum is opened with a sublabial antrostomy, the antral mucous membrane is removed, and an intranasal antrostomy made. The Caldwell-Luc operation, previously very commonly carried out, is now uncommon. Antibiotics and a possible change in the nature of the sinus disease account for this. If the ethmoid cells are involved, they can be removed with this approach (transantral ethmoidectomy). Chronic frontal sinusitis may also require surgery and is treated with an external approach. Obliteration of the sinus with a fat graft, or enlarging the fronto-nasal duct are the two current operations. The improvement of instruments and techniques for sinus endoscopy (page 40) has increased the possibilities of *sinus endoscopic surgery*. Biopsy of antral mucosa, excision of cysts and removal of foreign bodies (eg a misplaced apical dental filling) can be carried out via the sinus endoscope.

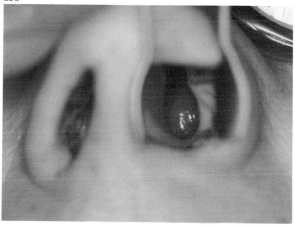

250 Nasal polyps These are a common cause of nasal obstruction, and may cause anosmia. They are benign and do not present with bleeding. Examination shows a grey pendulous opalescent swelling arising from the ethmoid. A polyp is very different in appearance from the red inferior turbinate adjacent to it.

Polyps may be solitary or multiple, often extending from the nasal vestibule to the posterior choana. They are usually bilateral. If ignored, nasal polyps may become extremely large, causing expansion of the nasal bones and alae nasi. A nasal polyp which is ulcerated and bleeds is probably malignant.

Nasal polyps result from a distension of an area of nasal mucous membrane with intercellular fluid. They are due to a hypersensitivity reaction in the mucous membrane, but may also result from sinus infection. Obstruction of the sinuses by polyps, however, may lead to a secondary sinusitis, and a sinus X-ray is a routine investigation.

Small nasal polyps may cause little in the way of symptoms and be chance-findings: usually, however, polyps extend and enlarge and present with nasal obstruction. They do regress with corticosteroid nose drops and sprays but in many instances surgical removal either under local or general anaesthesia is necessary.

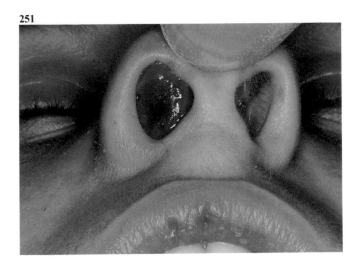

251 Nasal polyp extruding through the anterior nares. Large nasal polyps prolapse into the nasal vestibule with the exposed surface losing the opalescent grey colour and taking on the appearance of a carcinoma or papilloma.

252 Extensive nasal polyps which are ignored eventually expand the nasal bones and the external deformity of the nose and face may become gross. Surgical removal of the polyps may suffice in the elderly in whom this complication is usually seen. In the young, however, (**253,254**) rhinoplasty is also required to restore a normal nasal appearance.

252

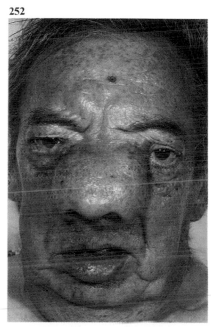

253

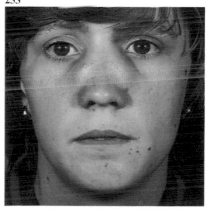

254

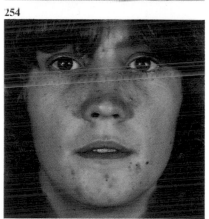

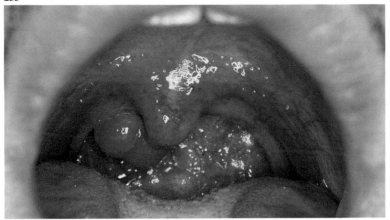

255 Nasal polyps in the oropharynx Extensive nasal polyps may extend beyond the soft palate and present in the oropharynx.

256 Enlarged posterior ends of the inferior turbinates Turbinates may enlarge in chronic rhinitis (and in nasal allergy) to produce a large polypoid mass obstructing the posterior choanae (*arrowed*). If these cannot be seen with the post-nasal mirror, they are demonstrated on the lateral X-ray.

256

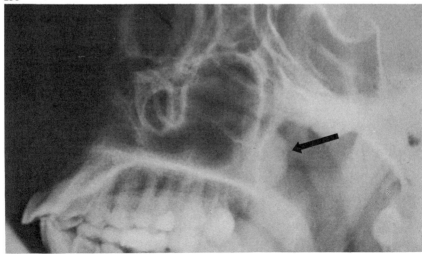

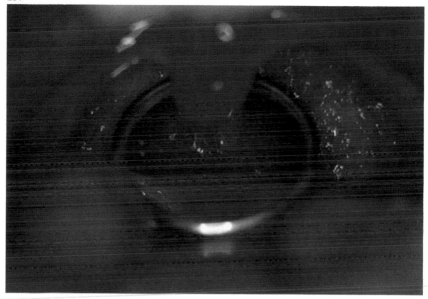

257 Antrochoanal polyp This is a special type of nasal polyp occurring in *adolescents* and young adults. Unilateral nasal obstruction is caused by a grey single polyp seen in the post-nasal space. The maxillary sinus is opaque on X-ray. A large antrochoanal polyp presents below the soft palate and extends into the oropharynx (**255**). A solitary polyp in one choana is almost certainly an antrochoanal polyp but a rare vascular polyp that should be remembered as a differential diagnosis is the *angiofibroma of male puberty*.

258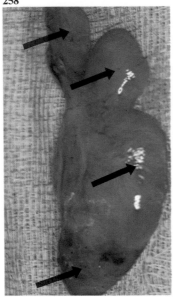

259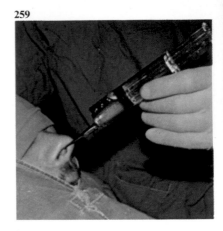

258 Antrochoanal polyp This type of polyp, which arises from the antral mucosa, extrudes through the ostium to fill the posterior nasal fossa and post-nasal space. It frequently becomes extremely large and extends below the soft palate. Removal of the polyp from its origin in the antrum through a sublabial antrostomy approach is necessary. The polyp is dumb-belled in shape with a pedicle connecting the nasal and antral portions. Intranasal removal is invariably followed by recurrence but may be necessary in early adolescence if the permanent dentition is endangered by a sublabial antrostomy. *Top arrow* shows polyp removed from antrum; *second arrow* shows polyp from nasal fossa; *third arrow* indicates polyp from post-nasal space; *bottom arrow* indicates polyp that has extended into oropharynx.

259 Aspiration from the antrum This shows straw-coloured fluid, and is a reliable diagnostic test for an antrochoanal polyp.

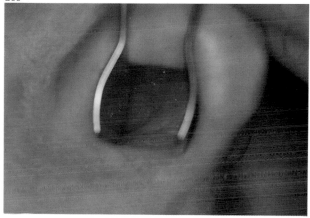

261

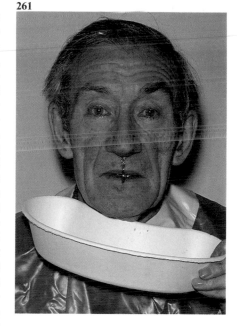

260,261 Epistaxis Anteriorly on the septum there is an anastomosis of several arteries (the sphenopalatine, the greater palatine, the superior labial and the anterior ethmoidal). This site is called Little's area or Kiesselbach's plexus and is the commonest site of nose bleeds. Although associated with alarm most epistaxis is short-lived and trivial. Firm pressure with the finger on the lateral wall of the nose opposite Little's area on the side of the bleeding, if maintained for about 4 minutes, will control the bleeding. It is better to sit upright, for the blood tends to be swallowed causing nausea on lying down. There are numerous causes of epistaxis. Some, such as trauma and acute inflammatory nasal conditions are obvious and common, but the more serious local and general causes must not be overlooked. Diagnosis must follow control of the epistaxis. Hypertension and blood dyscrasia are important general causes; neoplasms and telangiectasia may be underlying local factors.

151

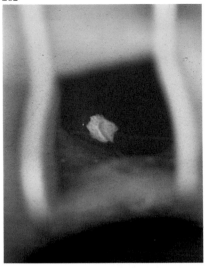

262 Cautery If epistaxis is recurrent, cautery (which is painless with local anaesthetic) to the bleeding point is necessary either with the galvano-cautery or with a chemical (eg trichloracetic acid or silver nitrate). Trichloracetic acid used in this case causes the bleeding site in Little's area to become white. Care must be taken to avoid the chemical running on to the skin of the vestibule or face as scarring will result. A topical anaesthetic is applied to the nasal mucous membrane in Little's area for galvano-cautery but, with silver nitrate and trichloracetic acid, no anaesthetic is needed and the procedure is painless, providing the vestibular skin is not touched.

263

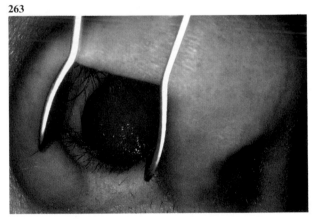

263 Hereditary nasal telangiectasia Frequent and often severe epistaxis is characteristic of this condition in which numerous leashes of bleeding vessels are apparent over Little's area of the nasal septum (and to be seen elsewhere, eg the hands, over the trunk). Cautery may be effective in the early stages but this condition is difficult to manage and may require extensive skin grafting on the nasal septum replacing the vascular septal mucosa, or oestrogen therapy.

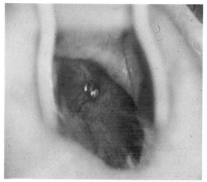

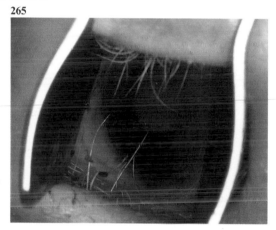

264,265 'Bleeding polyp Occasionally, a vascular sessile polyp is seen on the septum (haemangioma) which is the cause of severe recurrent bleeds. Treatment is excision, or cautery if the lesion is small.

Epistaxis from the anterior septum may be profuse and alarming but firm sustained pressure on the nares is invariably effective. Posterior epistaxis from the sphenopalatine artery may be very severe and difficult to manage. Nasal packing is needed to control the acute phase and ligation of the maxillary or external carotid artery is necessary if bleeding is persistent or severe. The terminal branch of the anterior ethmoidal artery may be the site of bleeding superiorly in the nose, particularly with nasal fractures: this vessel may require ligation. Recent radiographic techniques enable embolism of the terminal vessels to be carried out via an arterial catheter and is an option in managing very severe epistaxis, which may become life-threatening.

Neoplasms

Malignant nasal tumours A nasal polyp that does not appear grey and opalescent should arouse suspicion, as should a polyp that bleeds spontaneously. A solid-looking hyperaemic polyp may be a transitional cell papilloma. Granulation tissue in the nose may be malignant granuloma or carcinoma, and biopsy of any suspicious nasal lesion is necessary.

266   A pigmented polyp may be a malignant melanoma.

267-269   Carcinoma of the antrum or ethmoid These may extend not only into the nasal fossa and cheek (**267**) but may present in the oral cavity (**268**) appearing as a dental lesion. The antrum is opaque on X-ray with evidence of *bony destruction* (*arrowed*, **269**).

Prognosis when radiotherapy is followed by maxillectomy is quite good for an early maxillary carcinoma, but poor when there is extensive invasion. Exenteration of the orbit with maxillectomy is necessary when the eye is involved, but carcinoma with posterior spread to the base of the skull is inoperable. The use of cytotoxic drugs results in regression in some of these paranasal sinus neoplasms and is a further line of treatment. Extension of a neoplasm superiorly into the anterior cranial fossa involves resection superiorly of the dura and involved frontal lobe of the brain in continuity with the nasal and sinus neoplasm (**cranio-facial resection**).

266

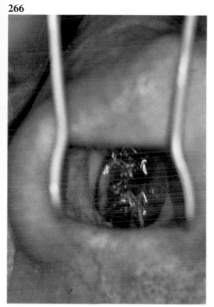

267

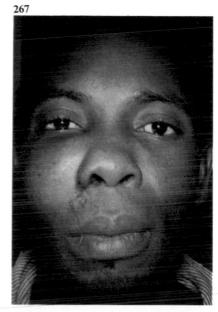

268

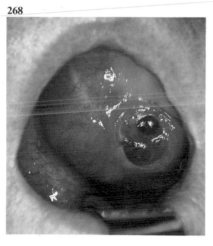

269

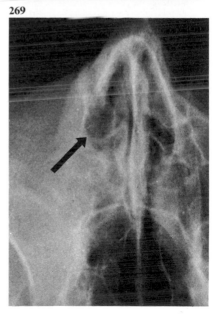

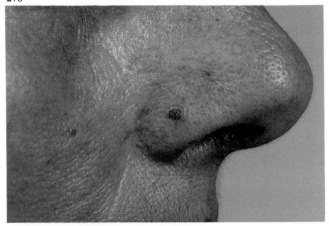

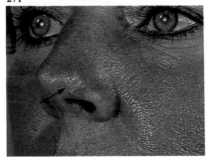

270,271 Basal cell carcinoma of nose One should be suspicious of an apparently innocent but chronic skin lesion which slowly increases in size. Excision with a good margin is curative. If, however, these lesions are ignored—and frequently they are disguised with cosmetics for months and even years—their excision can present considerable problems of reconstruction to avoid deformity in such an obvious site as the region of the nasal tip. Basal cell carcinomas in the groove at the base of the alae tend to erode deeply. Radiotherapy is the alternative treatment to surgery and with modern super-voltage therapy, lesions overlying cartilages can be treated with minimal risk of perichondritis.

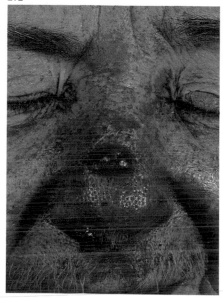
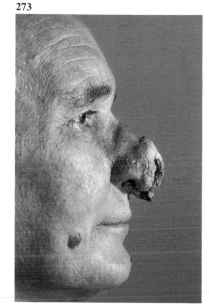

272   Carcinoma of the nose The apex of the nasal vestibule must be examined extremely carefully in a case of scanty epistaxis where no obvious bleeding site is apparent. Minimal bleeding and occasional sero-sanguineous discharge were this patient's presenting complaints. Later the carcinoma became obvious having eroded through the skin of the dorsum of the nose. Treatment with radiotherapy in this case was curative. Wide surgical excision with reconstruction of the nose was the alternative treatment.

273   Carcinoma of the external nose This is uncommon. Wide surgical excision with forehead reconstruction rhinoplasty, or less commonly radiotherapy are the available treatments.

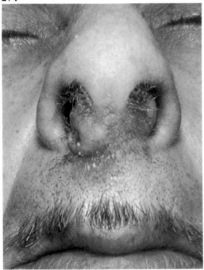

274 Carcinoma of the septum and columella

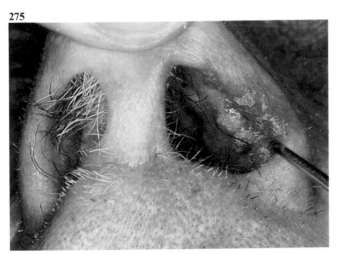

275 **Squamous cell carcinoma of the nasal vestibule** The history was short and the differential diagnosis of a basal cell carcinoma was made at biopsy.

276

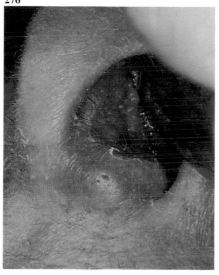

277

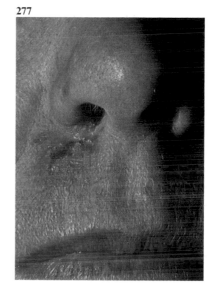

276 Carcinoma of the nasal septum
A biopsy of this ulcer on the septum and columella which presented with scanty epistaxis confirmed squamous cell carcinoma.

278

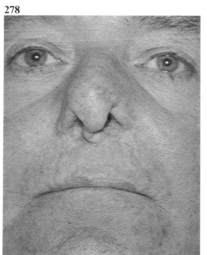

277 Chronic inflammation of the nose Lupus vulgaris is now rare. It presents as a chronic ulcer of the nasal vestibule extending on to the face. The differential diagnosis of inflammatory ulceration anteriorly in the nose includes **sarcoidosis** which may also cause destruction of the ala. Biopsy is necessary for the diagnosis.

278 The effects of lupus vulgaris Lupus, if ignored, is destructive to the skin and cartilage of the alae nasi and septum.

Symptoms of carcinoma of nasopharynx

Nasal
Obstruction
Sanguineous discharge

Neurological
Facial pain or
numbness due
to involvement
of Vth nerve

Ear
Deafness due to
secretory otitis media
Pain

Eye
Proptosis due to direct
spread to orbit
Diplopia due to involve-
ment of VIth nerve

Neck
Neck mass due to
cervical metastasis

279   Carcinoma of the nasopharynx This is uncommon in most countries but has an unexplained high incidence in the Far East, particularly in China, and East Africa.

There are many presenting symptoms (**279**). As the posterior choanae are large, nasal obstruction is not common with ulcerated carcinomas, which tend to present with symptoms of nerve involvement or secretory otitis media due to interference with the Eustachian tube. Lymphosarcomas and papilliferous carcinomas, however, cause obstruction. Carcinoma invades the skull base involving the Vth, VIth and Vidian (pterygoid) nerves, and may cause headache by invasion of the dura. The nasopharynx is a relatively concealed site and presentation of carcinoma is commonly late, with a cervical node metastasis.

The treatment is with radiotherapy. The overall prognosis is not good with about a 30 per cent five-year survival rate: this is, however, mainly related to the late diagnosis. An awareness of the early presenting symptoms and signs is essential for improved prognosis.

The Pharynx and Larynx

The oropharynx

280

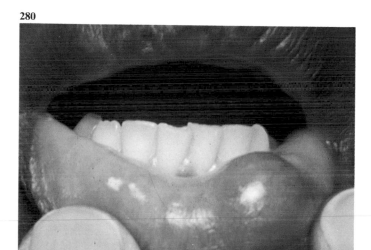

280 A mucocele of the lip Mucoceles are cystic, non-tender swellings presenting on the lips or in the oral cavity. They result from extravasation of mucus from a mucous gland into the surrounding tissue. Treatment is excision which is not always easy because of the extremely thin wall, and simple marsupialisation is often adequate.

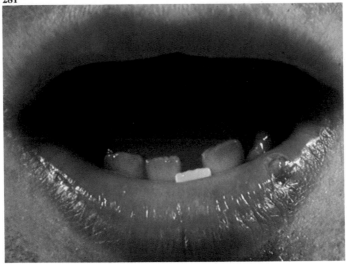

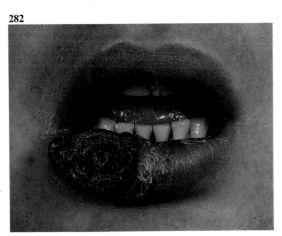

281,282 Lip ulcers Lip ulceration has numerous causes, either traumatic, inflammatory, or neoplastic: the provisional diagnosis can be made from the history and type of ulcer. Biopsy is necessary to confirm the diagnosis. The lesion is a *pyogenic granuloma*. Although these lesions are frequently small and related to trauma, they may enlarge from secondary infection (**282**) and take several weeks to heal.

283

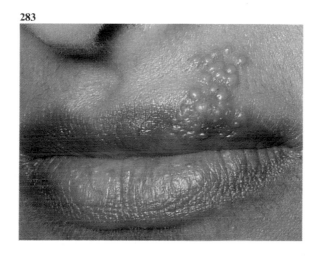

284

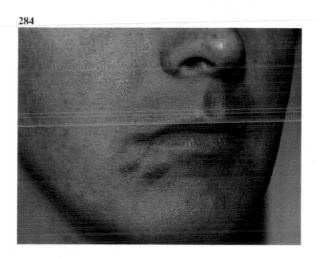

283,284 Herpes simplex of the lip showing the characteristic vesicles which later crust (**284**).

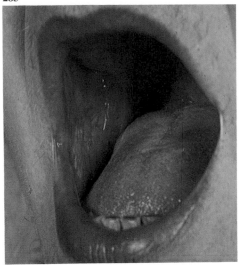

285 Keratosis may extend from the angle of the mouth along the occlusal plane of the teeth and is commonly a dental problem: it may be self-induced due to nervous cheek-biting. It is often the result of persistent trauma to the mucous membrane. When occurring in a site not exposed to trauma, eg the retromolar fossa, it should arouse suspicion that the mucosal change may be malignant and a biopsy is necessary.

286

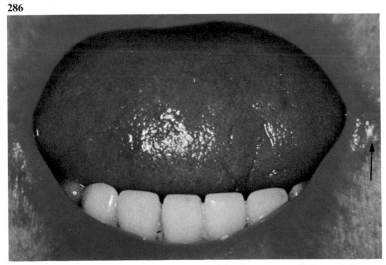

286 Angular stomatitis This occurs with the type of dental hyperkeratosis shown in **285**, but it may also be part of the Plummer-Vinson or Patterson-Brown-Kelly syndrome in which glossitis, seen here, and hypochromic anaemia are associated with a post-cricoid lesion, either a web or a carcinoma. This syndrome occurs mostly in women.

287

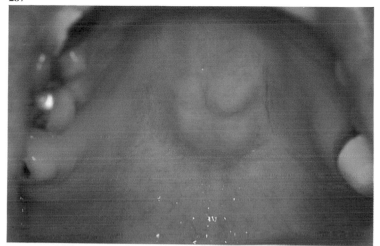

288

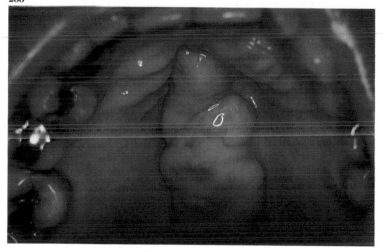

287,288 **The torus palatinus** The bony hard midline palatal swelling can be diagnosed confidently by its characteristics. It is a common finding and only requires removal if it interferes with the fitting of a denture. A large torus palatinus may take on a curious irregular appearance, suspicious of a carcinoma (**288**). Similar bony swellings occur on the lingual surface of the lower alveolus opposite the pre-molars (torus mandibularis).

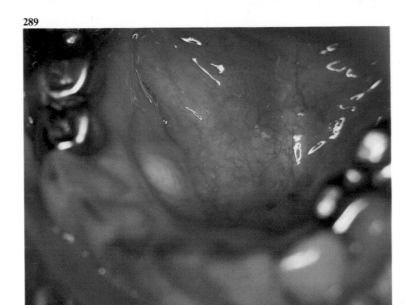

289   Torus mandibularis A white bony hard lesion arising from the inner aspect of the mandible may present as a swelling in the floor of the mouth. This is considerably less common than the torus palatinus.

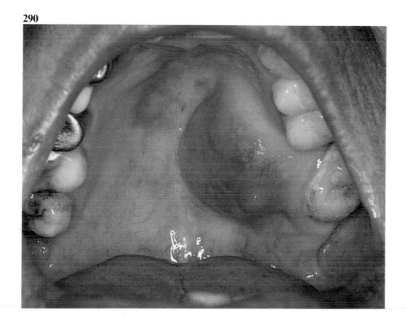

290 Ectopic pleomorphic adenoma A palatal swelling which is not bony and hard may be a fissural cyst if midline, but if placed to one side (as here), it is almost certainly a tumour of one of the minor salivary glands. Biopsy is necessary. It is frequently a pleomorphic adenoma, but may be an adenoid cystic carcinoma or other malignant salivary tumour. A tumour extension from the maxillary antrum must also be excluded.

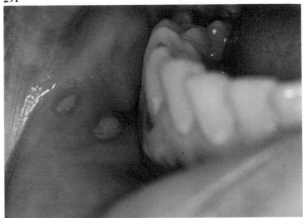

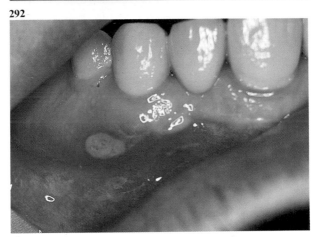

291,292 Aphthous ulcers An area of white superficial ulceration is surrounded by a hyperaemic mucous membrane. These commonly occur in crops of two or more and heal spontaneously in about one week. They are acutely tender and affect the non-keratinised oral mucous membrane. Although there is no induration on palpation, the histological inflammatory changes are not superficial and may extend into the underlying muscle.

Hydrocortisone pellets to suck, or triamcinolone with Orabase ointment applied to the ulcer are the most effective present treatments to relieve the pain. As the aetiology of these extremely common ulcers remains unknown, treatment is empirical.

293

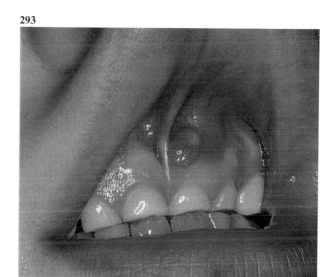

293 An aphthous-like ulcer overlying the apex of this deciduous tooth suggests the diagnosis of an apical dental abscess.

294

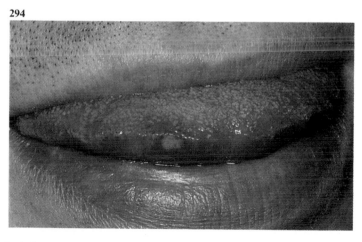

294 Aphthous ulcers on the tongue margin are often traumatic from tooth irregularity.

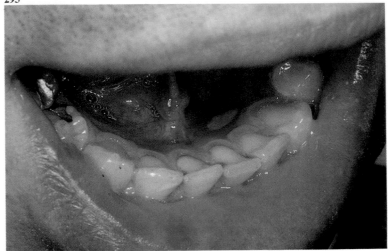

295   Trauma from a denture This may be an irritating factor, as may any minor trauma to the mucous membrane in a person susceptible to aphthous ulcers.

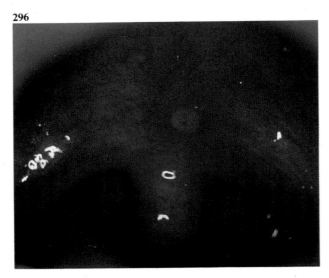

296   Aphthous ulcers are not uncommon on the soft palate.

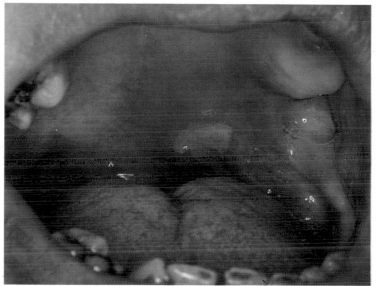

297 Solitary aphthous ulcer This ulcer (periadenitis mucosa necrotica recurrens) looks similar to a simple aphthous ulcer and is the same histologically, but it behaves differently. It is less common, larger, persists for several weeks or months and may leave a scar; it occurs in more varied sites affecting the soft palate and even the pyriform fossa, where it presents with severe dysphagia. Carbenoxolone ('Bioral') is used topically for the lesions in the oral cavity.

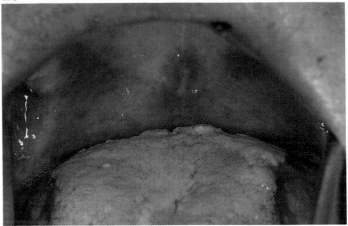

298 Multiple oral ulcers These may be the herpetiform type of aphthous ulceration but may be caused by a blood dyscrasia; if the ulcers are crusted and haemorrhagic the condition is either erythema multiforme or pemphigus. An iritis and genital ulceration may be present (Behçet's syndrome). High doses of systemic steroids are usually needed to control this type of severe ulceration. The snail-track ulcers of secondary syphilis must be remembered also in the differential diagnosis of oral ulceration (see **351**).

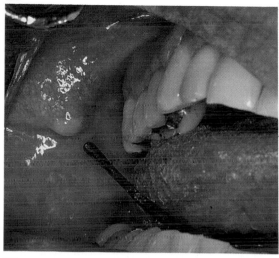

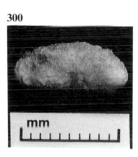

301

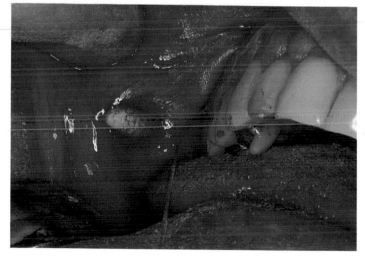

299—301 Parotid salivary calculus An ulcer in the region of the orifice of the parotid duct (**299**) suggests a possible salivary calculus. Parotid calculi are considerably less common than those in the submandibular duct but occasionally may occlude the orifice of the duct, causing painful intermittent parotid swelling, and require incision and removal (**300,301**).

The tongue

302

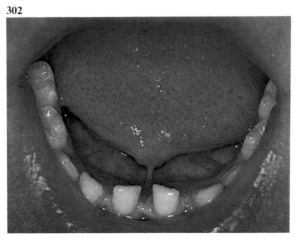

302 **'Tongue tie'** This is due to a short frenulum linguae, and apart from the defect of being unable to protrude the tongue, the patient is almost always symptom-free. Speech defects can rarely be attributed to tongue-tie necessitating division of the frenulum. Division is carried out under general anaesthetic and a suture may be required.

303

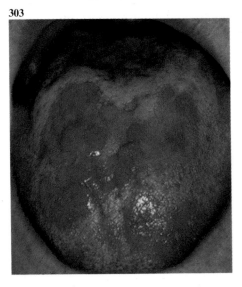

303 **Geographic tongue (benign migratory glossitis)** There are smooth areas with no filiform papillae. These areas vary in site on the tongue, and the appearance may concern the patient. It is, however, a condition of no significance requiring no treatment other than reassurance.

304

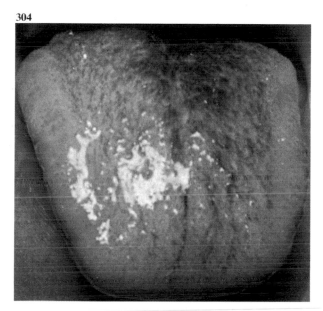

304 Black hairy tongue Patients not infrequently regard the appearance of their tongue as an index of their general health and are concerned to see a brown-black staining. This may be fungal (*Aspergillus niger*) and related to prolonged antibiotic therapy, but is frequently a chance finding with no other pathology than hypertrophy of the filiform papillae. Tobacco may be a cause. Scraping and cleaning the tongue temporarily improves the appearance but is unnecessary for this condition is harmless.

305 Haemangiomas of the tongue These may be chance findings and are usually innocuous. If large and giving rise to bleeding, laser surgery is the most effective present treatment.

305

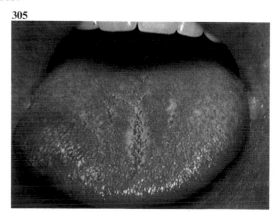

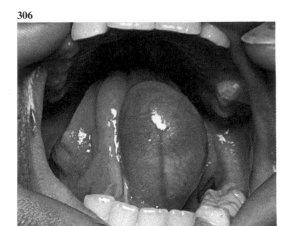

306 **The ranula** is a mucocele occurring in the floor of the mouth. A blue colour and the profunda vein stretched across the surface are characteristic. This ranula may extend into the tissues of the floor of the mouth and neck (plunging ranula). Total surgical removal is difficult because of the thin wall, and marsupialisation, as with the lip lesion (see **280**), is adequate treatment. Recurrence is not uncommon. The ranula may also present more in the floor of the mouth than on the undersurface of the tongue and the diagnosis may not be so obvious.

307

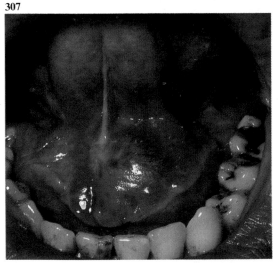

307 **A** **ranula** less well defined occupying the floor of the mouth.

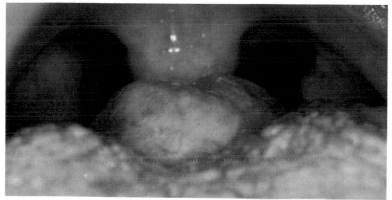

308 **Lingual thyroid** Developmental anomalies in the thyroid gland may result in thyroid tissue remaining at the foramen caecum or in the thyroglossal tract. The symptom-free swelling at the base of this tongue is thyroid tissue, and was shown on a radio-active iodine scan to be active. No thyroid gland was palpable in the neck and there was no iodine uptake other than at the base of the tongue. This lingual thyroid, therefore, was this patient's only active thyroid tissue.

309

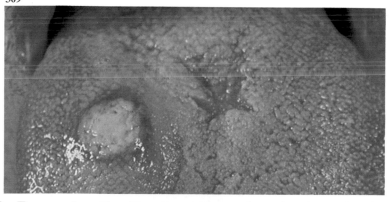

309 **Tongue ulceration** The site and type of tongue ulcers give the provisional diagnosis: a marginal ulcer with a raised edge is probably a carcinoma; an ulcer on the dorsum with a punched-out margin may be a gumma. Tuberculosis may be the cause of a tender ulcer of the tip of the tongue, in a country where tuberculosis is prevalent. These clinical findings are only guides, however, and biopsy of this ulcer on the dorsum showed it to be a solitary aphthous ulcer.

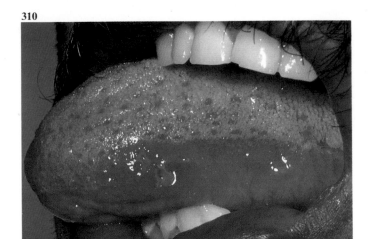

310 An aphthous tongue ulcer
311 Tongue ulceration from primary syphilis—a chancre

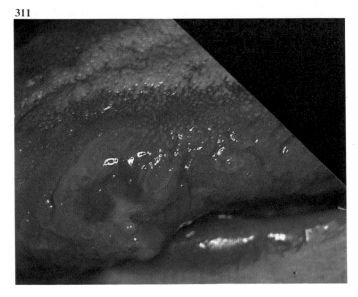

312 Laser excision of a tongue lesion showing the minimal reaction at the excision margin, and the non-bleeding base of the excision.

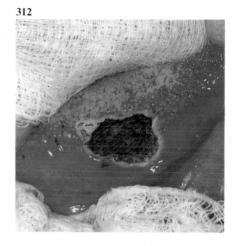

313 Median rhomboid glossitis This rare anomaly results from failure of the lateral halves of the tongue to fuse posteriorly, leaving the tuberculum impar in the midline. A smooth red, usually symptom-free area persists.

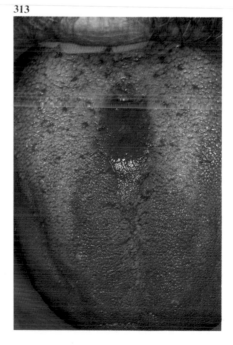

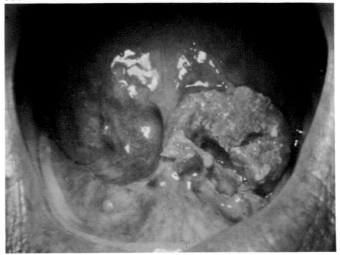

314 Carcinoma of the tongue This usually occurs on the margin or from the extension of an ulcer on the floor of the mouth (as shown here). Biopsy of this proliferative ulcer showed squamous cell carcinoma. Partial glossectomy in continuity with a neck dissection, or radiotherapy are the current treatments.

315

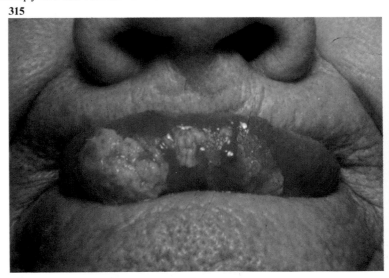

316

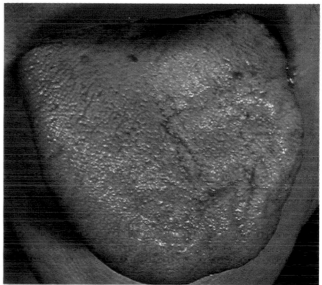

316 Hypoglossal nerve paralysis Initially there is fibrillation and later atrophy of the muscles on one side of the tongue. The tongue deviates on protrusion to the side of the nerve palsy. A destructive lesion in the region of the jugular foramen may extend to involve the hypoglossal nerve as it emerges from the nearby anterior condylar foramen. This paralysis of the tongue shows wrinkling caused by fibrillation, and is due to a glomus jugulare tumour, which has also damaged the cranial nerves that emerge through the jugular foramen (IX, X, and XI).

The hypoglossal nerve, if involved with cervical metastases, may be sectioned in the course of a radial neck dissection.

315 Leucoplakia This is precarcinomatous on the tongue. It may be secondary to dental or dietary irritation. Leucoplakia is also characteristic of tertiary syphilis, and the tongue is a site where the spirochaete predisposes to carcinoma. Leucoplakia, particularly with no apparent underlying traumatic cause, should be biopsied to exclude carcinoma.

317

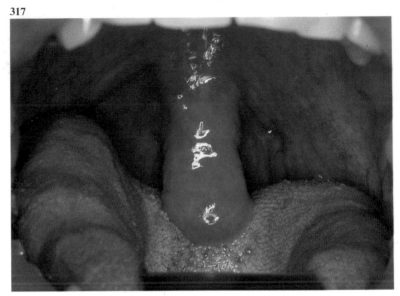

317 The uvula This obvious anatomical feature in the oropharynx has little pathological significance. When particularly long, however, as here, it has on occasions been thought responsible for various throat symptoms such as discomfort and snoring. Partial amputation has been recommended.

318 Bifid uvula A common minor congenital deformity of the palate. It is of little significance, but it may be associated with a submucous palatal cleft. Inflammation of the uvula, as an isolated entity may occur, however, and a cherry-like enlargement be the sole presenting sign of a sore throat

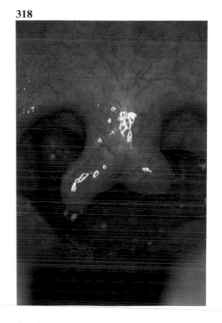

Snoring is probably rarely related solely to elongation of the uvula. Snoring is extremely common and in most cases tiresome but trivial and is accentuated by lesions causing obstruction in the upper respiratory tract. Snoring is conspicuous in children with obstruction from bulk of tonsillar and adenoid lymphoid tissue. The noise from snoring is produced from laxity and vibration of the oropharyngeal muscles. Obesity and excess alcohol are two relevant factors and frequently attention to these will reduce snoring. Gross snoring, however, may be associated with the *sleep apnoea syndrome* and when periods of apnoea occur at night with daytime somnolence, sleep studies are indicated. These may show significant variations in blood oxygen and CO_2 levels along with variations in cardiac and respiratory rates.

Cor pulmonale may occur in children with grossly obstructing tonsil and adenoid lymphoid tissue. Prolific adult snoring may require a *uvulopalatoplasty operation* in which the muscle and overlying mucosa of the palate and fauces are reduced, shortening the palate. The uvula is excised and the tonsils, if present, are removed. This treatment for snoring is indicated mainly when the snorer is at risk, rather than for the benefit of the one who listens.

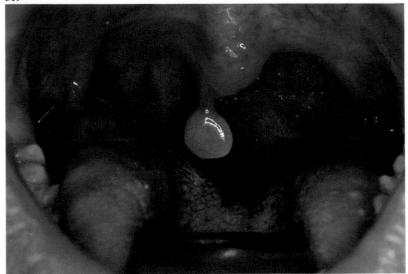

319 Papillomas These may occur on the uvula (**318**), the fauces and the tonsil. The patient often notices these papillomas when looking at the throat, or they are found at medical examination: symptoms are uncommon. They are usually pedunculated and are easily and painlessly removable in Outpatients. They should be sent for histology to exclude a squamous carcinoma. If ignored a papilloma may cause symptoms on account of size (**320**).

320

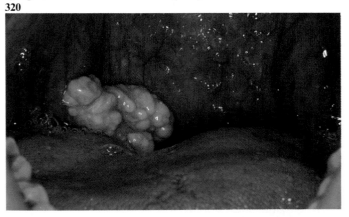

320   A large papilloma arising from the base of the right tonsil.

321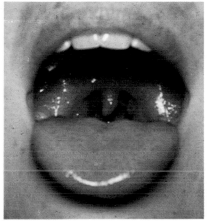

322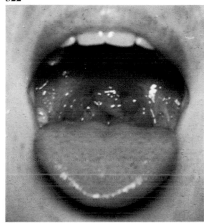

321,322 Tonsil size There is no recognised 'normal' size for a tonsil; it is, therefore, arguable whether tonsils can be described as 'enlarged'. The apparent size of the tonsil can be altered considerably when the tongue is protruded forcibly. This child, whose oropharynx looks normal with the tongue slightly protruded, can make the tonsils meet in the midline with maximum protrusion of the tongue.

323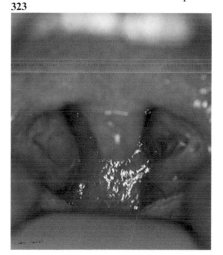

324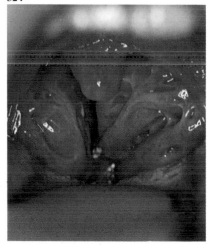

323,324 Tonsil size affected by tongue depressor The tongue depressor also alters the apparent size of the tonsils. If the tongue is firmly depressed, the patient gags and the tonsils meet in the midline.

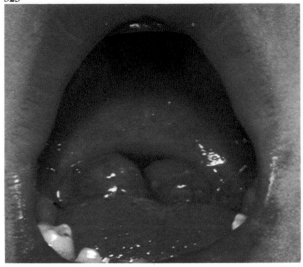

325,326 Tonsils meeting in the midline It is unusual, however, for the tonsils to meet in the midline or overlap, as in this case. Lymphoid tissue of this bulk, particularly during an acute tonsillitis, may cause respiratory obstruction and severe dysphagia. There is an increased awareness of the severity of upper respiratory tract obstruction from bulk of tonsillar and adenoid lymphoid tissue. In children, particularly at times of superimposed tonsillitis, the interference with breathing becomes alarming and obstructive sleep apnoea syndrome is now well-recognised as an important indication for surgery to remove the tonsils and adenoids. Cor pulmonale is seen in children with marked upper respiratory tract obstruction.

326

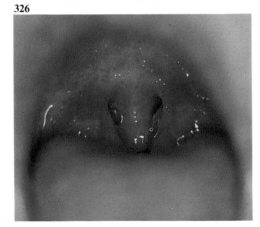

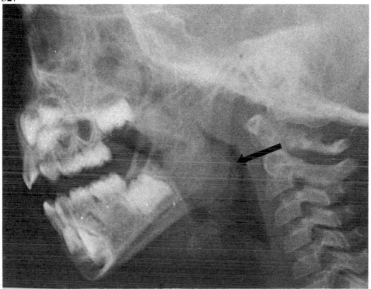

327 Lateral X-ray of tonsils The tonsils and adenoids show on lateral X-ray and the soft tissue shadow helps in assessing the degree of obstruction that the lymphoid tissue may be causing. The *lingual tonsil* is unusually large in Down's syndrome patients and contributes to their characteristic bulky tongue.

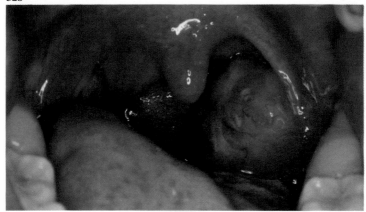

328 Unilateral tonsil enlargement A tonsil can be described as 'large' when compared with the other tonsil. A conspicuously large tonsil in the absence of acute inflammation is an important finding suggesting either a *chronic quinsy* or a *lymphosarcoma*. A persistent and conspicuously large tonsil, therefore, should be removed for histology.

329

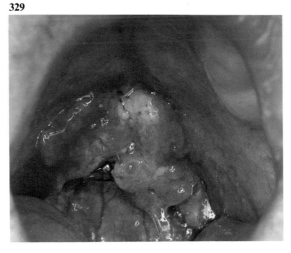

329 A palate and tonsil carcinoma This presents as an indurated ulcer rather than a diffuse enlargement, and causes pain and otalgia. The biopsy is taken from the ulcer margin. The five-year survival following radiotherapy is about 20 per cent.

330

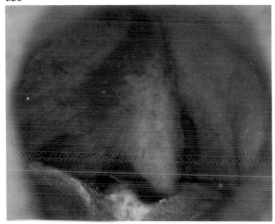

331

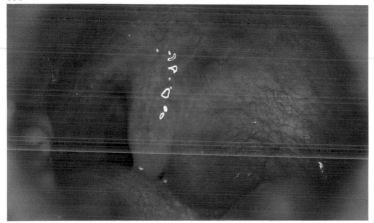

330,331 Simulated tonsil enlargement A tonsil may appear to be enlarged by *medial displacement* from a *parapharyngeal swelling* and careful examination of the fauces ensures that the correct diagnosis is made. It is possible to biopsy a normal tonsil and realise later that medial displacement is simulating enlargement. In this case (**330**) the parapharyngeal mass is an internal carotid aneurysm: the initial diagnosis in Casualty was a quinsy—a dangerous error if followed by incision. Other more common parapharyngeal swellings are tumours of the deep lobe of the parotid gland, (**331**), chemodectomas, neurofibromata and enlargement of the parapharyngeal lymph nodes.

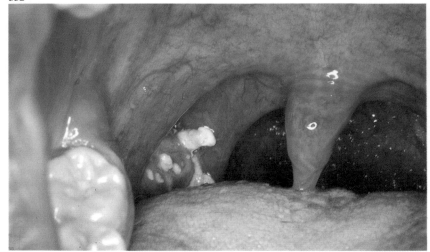

332,333 Keratosis pharyngeus Yellow spicules due to hyper-keratinized areas of epithelium are sometimes extensive over the tonsil and lingual tonsil. It is usually a chance finding, and it is important in diagnosis to probe the tonsil to be certain that these yellow areas are not exudate. No treatment is required for this condition unless it is associated with tonsillitis.

333

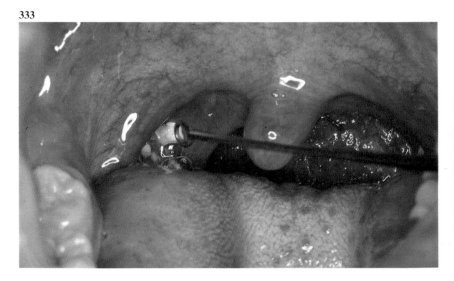

334

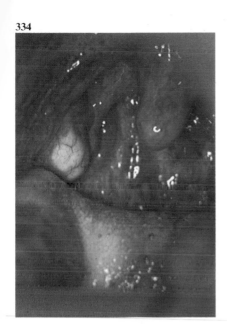

334,335 Retention cysts These are common on the tonsil and appear as sessile yellow swellings. If small, they can be ignored and although symptoms are uncommon, a concern by the patient or a sensation of a lump in the throat, may call for surgical removal. Retention cysts are also seen following tonsillectomy in the region of the fauces (**335**).

335

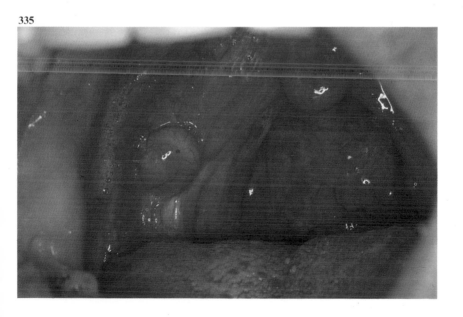

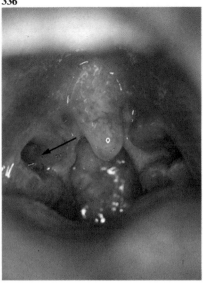

336 Supratonsillar cleft This recess near the superior pole of the tonsil tends, if large, to collect debris. A mass of yellow fetid material can be extruded from the tonsil with pressure, and discomfort or *halitosis* are symptoms with which this condition may present. Tonsillectomy may be necessary. The surgeon, however, must beware of tonsillectomy for halitosis. Although dental or gastric pathology may cause this symptom, as may a pharyngeal pouch, the symptom may be imagined by the patient, or in the mind of the other person complaining about the halitosis.

337

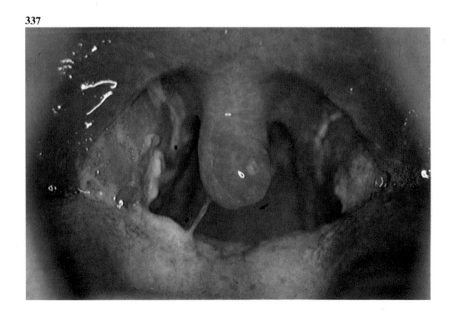

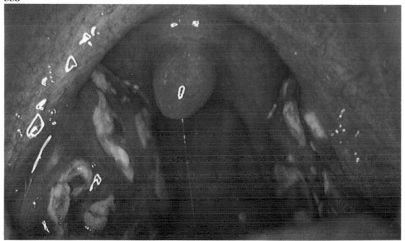

337,338 Acute tonsillitis This condition is characterised by sore throat, dysphagia and pyrexia. The appearance of the tonsils varies: an obviously purulent exudate covering the tonsils is common and is either diffuse (**337**) or punctate (**338**). An apparently less severely infected throat, with only hyperaemia of the tonsils, however, may be associated with severe symptoms. The tonsillar lymph nodes near the angle of the mandible are large and tender.

With acute tonsillitis the exudate and hyperaemia are centred on the tonsils: in an acute pharyngitis, as may be associated with a head cold, the mucous membrane of the entire oropharynx is hyperaemic. The gonococcus may cause acute pharyngitis and a throat swab must be placed in Stewart's medium for laboratory examination if this infection is suspected. The throat swab in acute tonsillitis commonly grows the haemolytic streptococcus, and a course of oral penicillin (often supplemented with an initial intramuscular injection) is invariably curative. An analgesic may also be needed, but lozenges and gargles are usually unnecessary.

339

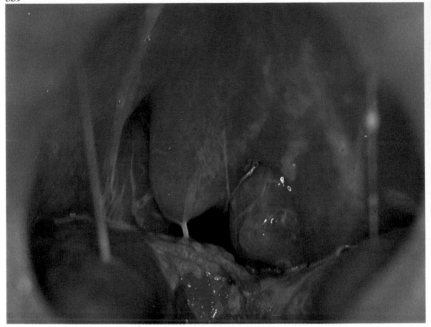

340

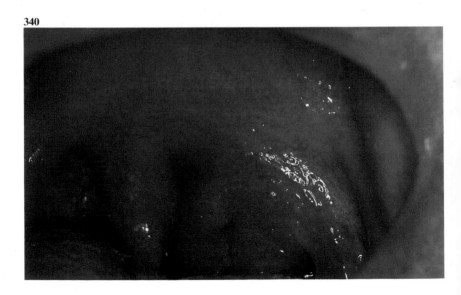

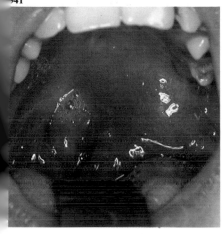 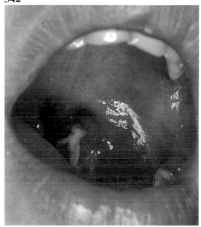

339-342 A quinsy This is a complication of acute tonsillitis in which a peritonsillar abscess forms. The symptoms may be extremely severe with absolute dysphagia, pain referred to the ear and trismus. There is malaise, fever and marked swelling of the tonsillar lymph node. Examination shows the signs of acute tonsillitis with medial displacement of the tonsil to the midline.

If the abscess is pointing, incision at the site marked releases the pus. Since the advent of antibiotics the need for incision of quinsies is less. High doses of intramuscular penicillin for five days is the treatment and should be followed by a further five-day course of oral penicillin. A large tonsil with medial displacement persists with inadequate treatment and represents a chronic quinsy in which recurrence of an acute episode is common. A throat swab of the pus is taken at the time of diagnosis and the result may later require the penicillin to be changed to another antibiotic.

A quinsy is extremely rare in children and is also rarely bilateral. Complications are uncommon, but *bleeding* from a quinsy is an important and serious sign: it is due to erosion by the peritonsillar pus of one of the adjacent vessels—either one of the tonsillar arteries or the internal carotid artery (**bleeding quinsy**). Quinsies not infrequently occur in those who have suffered previous episodes of acute tonsillitis. Tonsillectomy, which is indicated after a quinsy, is delayed four to six weeks until the acute phase has passed. Vascular fibrous tissue found lateral to the tonsil after a quinsy makes tonsillectomy technically difficult and some advocate tonsillectomy at the time of the acute quinsy (**quinsy tonsillectomy**).

343

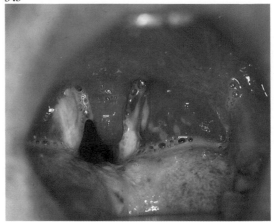

344

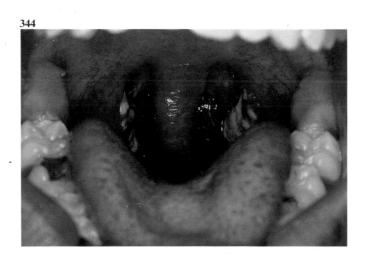

345

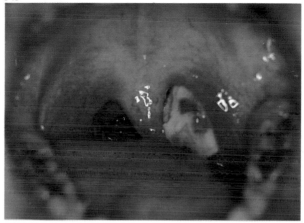

346

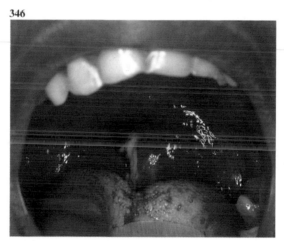

343-346 **Infectious mononucleosis** *This should be suspected if a sore throat and malaise persist despite antibiotic treatment, and a white cell analysis and Paul-Bunnell are indicated.* A white membrane covering one or both tonsils is characteristic and helpful in diagnosis. Hypersensitivity to ampicillin is increased in infectious mononucleosis and the antibiotic should be avoided: a severe urticaria follows its use. The positive Paul-Bunnell blood test is diagnostic of infectious mononucleosis, and atypical mononuclear white cells are increased on the blood film.

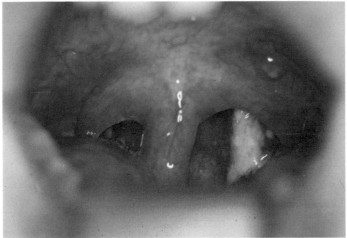

347 Infectious mononucleosis in a patient without tonsils In this case
the membrane characteristic of infectious mononucleosis is seen
either on the lingual tonsil or, as in this case, on a *prominent posterior
pharyngeal band of lymphoid tissue*. A similar white membrane also
covers the lymphoid tissue in the post-nasal space and the appearance
on examination of the post-nasal space is suspicious of neoplasm. The
increase in bulk of the adenoids also caused a 'nasal voice', which is
sometimes characteristic of infectious mononucleosis.

348

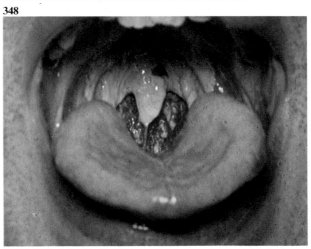

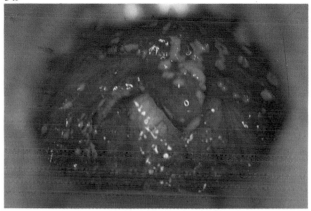

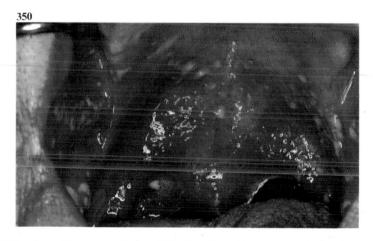

348-350 **Monilia or oral candidiasis (thrush)** is one of the fungal infections of the pharynx. Extensive white areas cover the entire oropharynx, and are not confined to the tonsil. They are either continuous (**348**) or punctate (**349**): a swab shows *Candida albicans* and confirms the diagnosis. The condition responds to antifungal mouth washes or lozenges containing nystatin or amphotericin. It is commoner in neonates, and may complicate treatment with broad spectrum antibiotics. Oral candidiasis is one of the commonest upper respiratory tract manifestations of AIDS; unexplained oral fungal infection should make the possibility of AIDS a diagnostic consideration (**350**). Nasal vestibulitis and cervical lymphadenopathy may be associated findings.

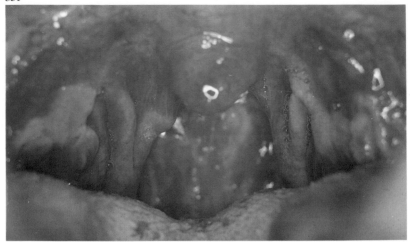

351 Ulcers on the tonsil and soft palate *Candida* was cultured, but these are *snail-track ulcers of secondary syphilis*.

352

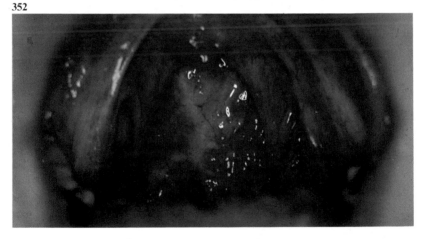

352 Chronic pharyngitis In this condition there is a generalised hyperaemia of the pharyngeal mucous membrane, with hyperaemic masses of lymphoid tissue on the posterior wall of the oropharynx. A persistently slight sore throat is the main symptom. The cause is usually 'irritative' rather than due to chronic infection; environment and occupation, diet and tobacco are the common factors.

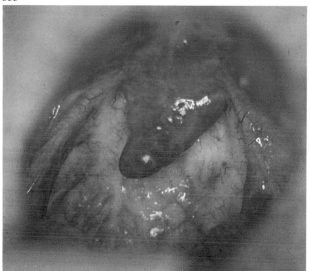

353 Scleroma with scarring of the soft palate and oropharynx This is a specific chronic inflammatory disease of the upper respiratory tract mucosa predominantly occurring in Eastern Europe, Asia and South America. A protracted painless inflammation of the nose (**rhinoscleroma**), pharynx, or larynx is followed after many years by extensive scarring, which is particularly apparent in the oropharynx. Unlike gummatous ulceration, which is a differential diagnosis, scleroma is not destructive, and the uvula is preserved, although it may be retracted by scarring into the naso-pharynx, and seen with the post-nasal mirror. The histology of the mucosa in scleroma is characteristic and diagnostic.

Tonsillectomy

This is one of the most frequently performed operations in the world. More strict indications for operating, however, are reducing the number of tonsillectomies. Recurrent episodes of acute tonsillitis, interfering with school or work, are the main indications: a quinsy or chronic tonsillitis are other indications.

354

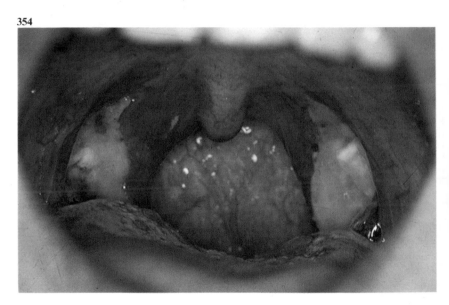

354 The tonsillar fossae following tonsillectomy These are covered with a white/yellow membrane for about ten days until the fossae are epithelialised.

355 Tonsils after removal to demonstrate the lingual pole (*arrow*) The pole must be included at tonsillectomy. A tonsil remnant may be left inadvertently at this site and give rise to further infection. Tonsils do not 'regrow'. Adenoid tissue, however, is not possible to enucleate and remove *in toto*; it may recur, particularly when removed before 4 years of age.

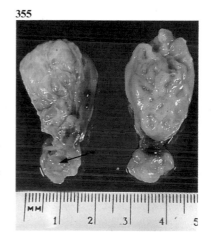

355

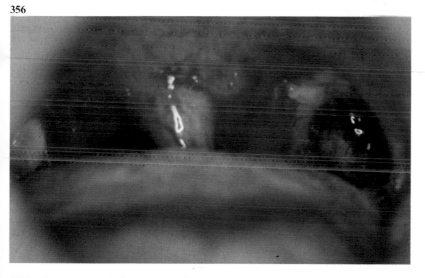

356

356 Secondary infection A blood clot in the tonsillar fossa is an important postoperative finding and almost certainly indicates secondary infection. This occurs between the third and tenth day and is associated with an increase in the pain, and bleeding. The bleeding is usually scanty and settles when antibiotics control the secondary infection. Severe delayed bleeding after tonsillectomy may occur, however, and the finding of a blood clot in a tonsillar fossa must not be ignored.

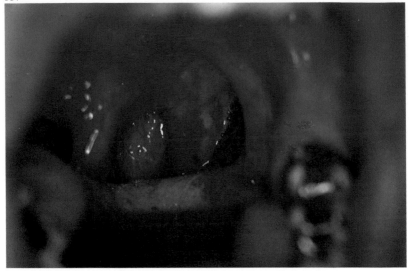

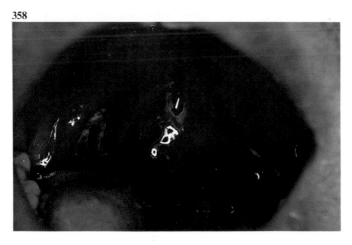

357,358 Secondary tonsillar infection with bleeding and bruising of the soft palate This appearance may be related to an excessively traumatic tonsillectomy. An infected blood clot is present in the tonsillar fossa: removal may cause more bleeding. A tonsillar blood clot present with primary bleeding, however, should be removed if possible and the bleeding may settle.

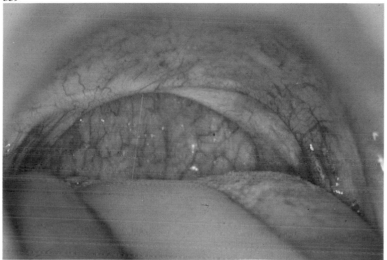

359 Guillotine tonsillectomy Tonsillectomy today is by dissection with minimal injury to the fauces and surrounding structures. Adept use of the guillotine may also be a rapid and effective surgical technique, but removal of the uvula and fauces is possible in inexperienced hands. Fortunately *postoperative scarring* of the palate and uvula is frequently symptom-free and this appearance of the soft palate with conspicuous shortening is similar to that following the **uvulopalatoplasty** operation for severe snoring.

Inflammation of the larynx

Laryngitis Whether acute or chronic, laryngitis presents with hoarseness and generalised hyperaemia of the laryngeal mucous membrane. Acute laryngitis commonly follows an upper respiratory tract infection, or is traumatic following vocal abuse (**367**). Voice rest is the most effective treatment. Chronic laryngitis may be associated with infection in the upper or lower respiratory tract, but is commonly 'irritative' due to occupation and environment, vocal abuse or tobacco. The unusual laryngitis of **myxoedema** must not be forgotten.

360

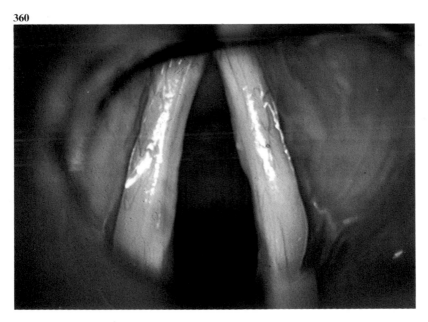

360 Normal vocal cords These are ivory coloured and smooth with few vessels on the surface. This is the view obtained through a laryngoscope at direct laryngoscopy.

361

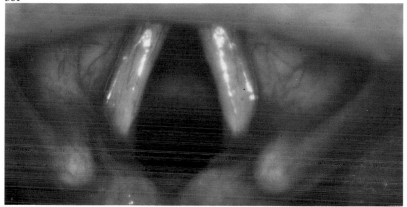

361   A fibreoptic endoscopic view of a normal larynx (see **58**)

362

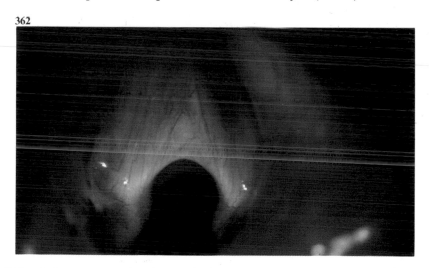

362   A laryngeal web Congenital abnormalities of the larynx are
uncommon. Webbing of varying degrees of severity is one of the
commoner developmental abnormalities, and present as hoarseness.
Similar webbing may follow inadvertent trauma at endoscopic surgery to *both* vocal cords near the anterior commissure. A mucosal
web is treated with surgical division. Most webs, however, are deep
and fibrous and need an indwelling 'kecl' after division to avoid recurrence.

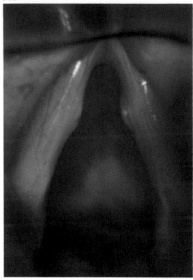

363 Laryngeal nodules A specific and localised type of chronic laryngitis, often seen in professional voice users, is *laryngeal nodules* (singers' nodules). Initially an oedema is seen on the vocal cord between the anterior one-third and posterior two-thirds of the cord. Removal of the nodules may be necessary, but attention to the underlying voice production by a speech therapist is the most important aspect of treatment. These nodules are not an uncommon cause of *hoarseness in children*, particularly of large families involved in competitive shouting ('screamers' nodules). Vocal cord nodules are also seen in those who over-use or misuse their voices.

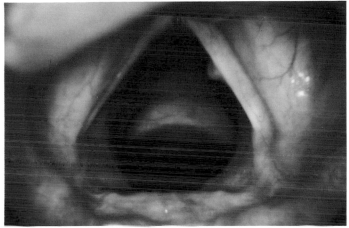

364 Vocal cord nodule seen through a fibreoptic endoscope
A solitary vocal cord nodule at the characteristic site is not uncommon, although they are usually bilateral and fairly symmetrical.

365 A vocal cord nodule with haematoma formation following vocal abuse.

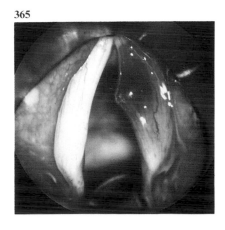

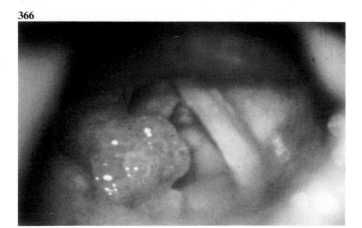

366 Juvenile papillomas are most important to exclude in a hoarse child, for if the hoarseness is ignored stridor will develop as the papillomas extend to occlude the lumen of the larynx. ('Screamers' nodules [laryngeal nodules], however, are the commonest cause of hoarseness in children.)

In this curious condition multiple wart-like excrescences develop, usually before the age of five, on or around the vocal cords. Recurrence follows removal but fortunately there is regression or a reduced rate of growth at adolescence. The cause is now established as the human papilloma virus. Management consists of regular microlaryngoscopy with removal of the papillomas using the carbon dioxide laser (or suction-diathermy). A tracheostomy may be necessary but should be avoided if possible as papillomas tend to develop around the tracheal opening and 'seed' further down the tracheobronchial tree. In severe cases chemotherapy with interferon is currently being evaluated.

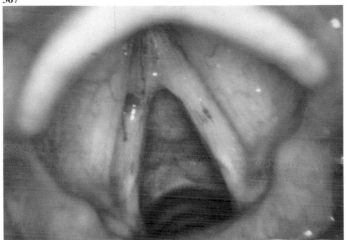

367 Acute laryngitis showing slight hyperaemia and oedema of both vocal cords seen with the fibreoptic endoscope.

368

369

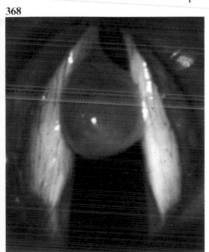

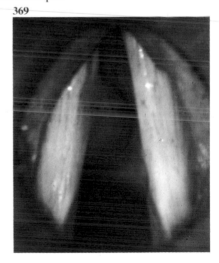

368,369 Pedunculated vocal cord polyp A large pedunculated polyp may form on the vocal cord and be missed on examination for it moves above and below the cord on expiration and inspiration. A large polyp (**368**) is less apparent (**369**) when it is below the cord on inspiration.

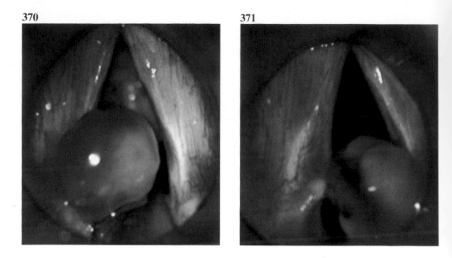

370,371 Intubation granulomas of the larynx These result from trauma by the anaesthetic tube to the mucosa overlying the vocal process of the arytenoid; they are, therefore, posterior. With the skill that anaesthetists have achieved for endotracheal intubation, trauma to this region is uncommon. Granulomas at this site also develop after prolonged vocal abuse has caused a chronic laryngitis in which the epithelium over the vocal process becomes ulcerated ('**contact ulcers**'). Removal at the pedicle is necessary. Figure **371** shows the pedicle of the intubation granuloma being held with forceps prior to removal. Recurrence frequently follows excision but laser beam techniques appear to lessen the likelihood. Relatively large lesions can occupy the posterior half of the larynx with minimal voice change. Anteriorly in the larynx, however, small lesions cause conspicuous voice change.

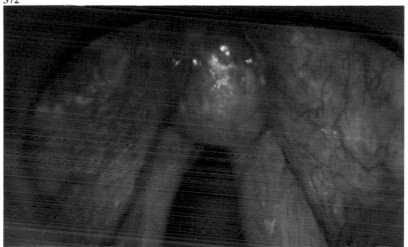

372 Polyp at the anterior commissure This is not always easy to see on indirect laryngoscopy for it may be partly obscured by the tubercle of the epiglottis. The laryngoscope is placed against the tubercle, displacing it forwards and a clear view is obtained.

373

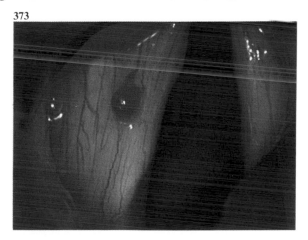

373 Haemangiomas These are uncommon vocal cord lesions and if small may cause no hoarseness or bleeding, and be a chance finding on examination. Laser surgery promises to be the effective treatment for larger haemangiomas.

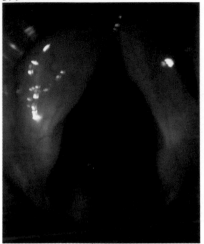

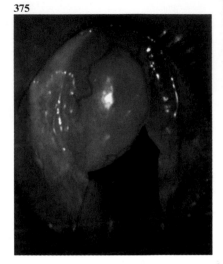

374,375 Chronic laryngitis With this condition hyperaemia of the mucous membrane may be associated with other changes in the larynx. Oedema of the margin of the vocal cords is common (Ranke's oedema), so that the free margin is polypoid and a large sessile polyp may form. The oedema, although affecting both cords, may be more marked on one side.

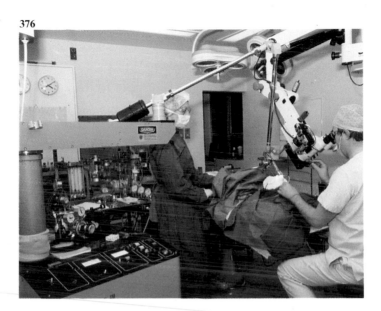

376 The laser The laser beam for surgical excision may prove to be the technique of choice for certain lesions in the upper respiratory tract. In this case it is being used at microlaryngoscopy to excise an intubation granuloma (page 212). The laser is now widely used for the removal of tongue (see **312**) and pharyngeal lesions, particularly haemangiomas and other vascular lesions. The laser also appears to have advantages for excision of juvenile papillomas, intubation granulomas and possibly laryngeal webs. Use of the operating microscope ensures precise excision with the laser beam, which causes considerably less tissue damage than cautery or diathermy.

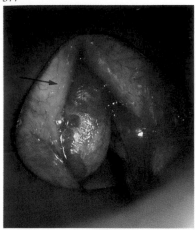

377 Hypertrophy of the ventricular bands is another finding in chronic laryngitis and they may meet in the midline on phonation, producing a characteristic hoarseness. Ranke's oedema is also present. Microlaryngoscopy and surgical excision of the oedematous margins is effective with dissection or the laser beam. Excision to the anterior commissure is made on one cord only to avoid webbing.

378

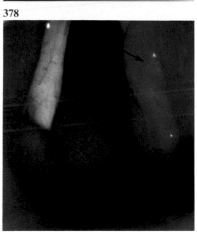

379

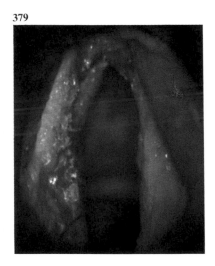

378 Prolapse of the ventricular mucous membrane This may also occur in chronic laryngitis and presents as a supraglottic swelling. A supraglottic cyst or carcinoma must be excluded.

379 Longstanding chronic laryngitis The mucous membrane may become extremely hypertrophic with white patches (leucoplakia). Histologically the white patches represent areas of keratosis which may precede malignant change and be reported as **carcinoma-in-situ**. This patient had smoked over sixty cigarettes a day for fifty years.

Neoplasms of the larynx

380

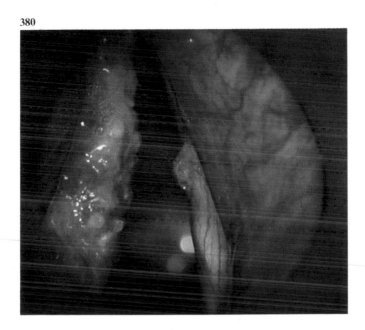

380 Carcinoma of the vocal cord This usually occurs in smokers. The indurated leucoplakia on this vocal cord is a well differentiated squamous cell carcinoma that has arisen as a result of chronic laryngitis with hyperkeratosis. The prognosis for vocal cord carcinoma with radiotherapy is excellent, with a cure rate of over 90 per cent for early lesions. The voice returns to normal, as does the appearance of the vocal cord.

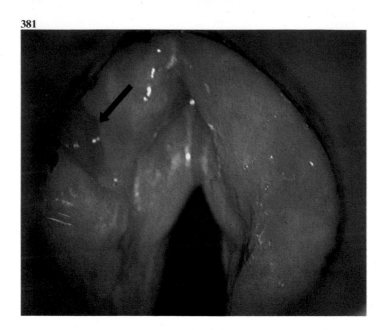

381 Supraglottic squamous cell carcinoma Carcinoma of the larynx commonly involves the vocal cord (glottic carcinoma), but lesions may develop below the cord (subglottic) or above the cord (supra-glottic). The ulcerated area of granulation tissue above the oedematous vocal cord in this case is a squamous cell carcinoma. The prognosis for supraglottic and subglottic carcinoma is worse than for glottic carcinoma, for hoarseness is delayed until the cord is involved and the greater vascularity and lymphatic drainage above and below the cord predisposes to earlier metastasis.

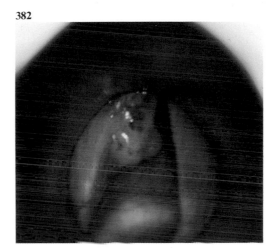

382 Subglottic carcinoma

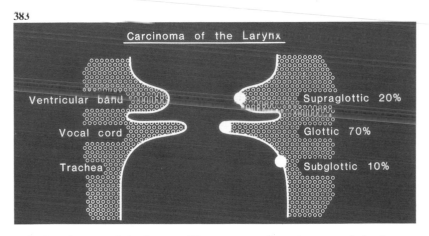

383 Carcinoma of the larynx 70 per cent of carcinomas of the larynx affect the vocal cord.

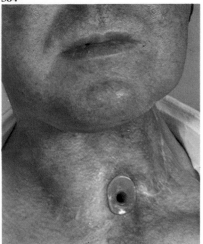

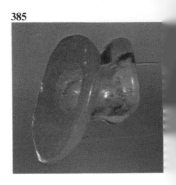

384 Total laryngectomy with left radical neck dissection Nearly all cases of early carcinoma of the vocal cord are cured with radiotherapy. Disease, however, may remain with extensive cord carcinomas, with supra or subglottic lesions, or with carcinoma of the pyriform fossa or epiglottis. **Partial laryngectomy** (laryngofissure, extended laryngofissure or supraglottic laryngectomy) gives adequate resection of some laryngeal carcinomas, but frequently a total laryngectomy is required. This radical surgery, which may be associated with a neck dissection if the nodes are involved, means a permanent tracheostome, and an alternative method of speech has to be developed. Air is swallowed into the upper oesophagus and coherent speech is achieved by learning to phonate with controlled regurgitation of the air. Even with intensive speech therapy some patients remain unable to achieve reasonable voice. Conservative laryngectomy (supraglottic or hemi-laryngectomy) aims in the smaller laryngeal cancers to preserve part or all of the vocal cords and avoid a tracheostome, so that laryngeal voice is preserved. For those who are unable to speak after total laryngectomy, or as a primary procedure with laryngectomy, a valve fitted between the tracheostome and oesophagus enables air to be redirected with a more normal voice production (Blom-Singer valve).

385 Stomal stud Stenosis of the tracheostome is sometimes a post-operative problem and a small stomal stud can be used.

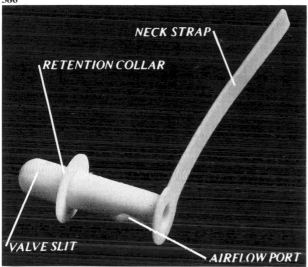

386, 387 The Blom-Singer voice prosthesis shown diagrammatically and positioned into the new opening to the oesophagus at the top of the tracheostome. This prosthesis may be inserted at the time of laryngectomy or placed later in those who are unable to develop coherent speech.

387

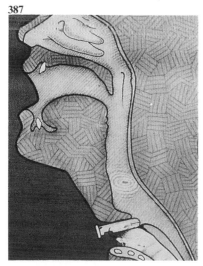

388

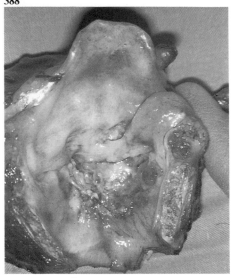

388 Laryngectomy specimen Shows a large laryngeal carcinoma extending above and below the right vocal cord and across to the left side of the larynx. It also shows the hyoid, thyroid and cricoid cartilages and upper rings of trachea, which are removed at laryngectomy.

389, 390 Laryngeal tomogram This (see **43**) is a helpful investigation for a larynx that is difficult or impossible to see on indirect examination. **389** shows an extensive carcinoma; **390** shows a large pedunculated supraglottic swelling, which proved to be a fibroma — a rare benign laryngeal tumour.

389

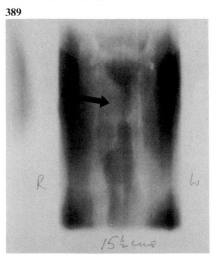

390

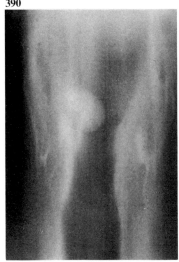

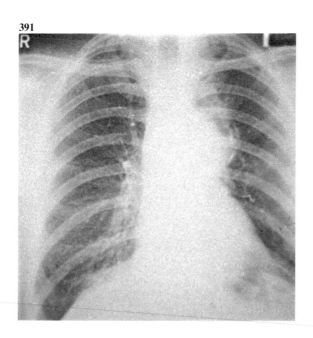

391 Secondaries from lung carcinoma Hoarseness may be due to **paralysis of one vocal cord**. Lack of cord movement on phonation is diagnosed on indirect laryngoscopy. Although temporary idiopathic cord palsy is the single most common cause, involvement of the left recurrent laryngeal nerve in chest disease must be excluded. Any hilar lymph node lesion in the region of the aortic arch may involve this nerve, such as secondaries from lung carcinoma. The enlarged left atrium of mitral stenosis may also press on the left recurrent laryngeal nerve and cause hoarseness, as may an aortic aneurysm or the enlarged pulmonary artery of pulmonary hypertension.

The recurrent laryngeal nerves are also occasionally damaged in the neck by severe external injury, or by thyroid carcinoma or by surgery. Central lesions, or lesions near the jugular foramen involving the vagus may also cause cord paralysis, and hoarseness is one of the symptoms of posterior inferior cerebellar artery thrombosis.

Hoarseness, particularly a whispered voice, with normal larynx is a functional voice problem. **Hysterical aphonia** is not uncommon in young women, and stems from a superficial psychiatric upset. Treatment from the speech therapist is usually effective without referral to a psychiatrist being necessary. Curious alterations in the voice or hoarseness may also be due to a **hysterical dysphonia.**

Microsurgery of the larynx

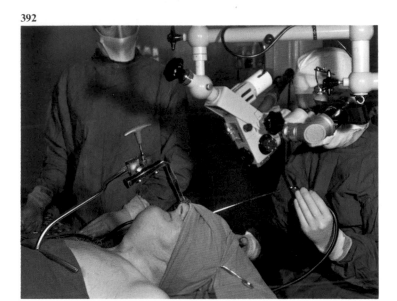

392, 393 Microlaryngoscopy The use of the microscope for direct laryngoscopy has greatly increased the scope and precision of laryngeal surgery. All small benign lesions of the larynx are better excised with this technique. Biopsies of malignant disease can be taken accurately from the suspicious area with minimal damage to adjacent tissue.

The holder for the laryngoscope is clamped and enables the surgeon to have both hands free for instrumentation. The X-rays are seen in the background (**393**): the chest X-ray and X-ray of the cervical spine are routine investigations before direct laryngoscopy. Cold light instruments give brighter and more reliable illumination than bulbs, and the development of a light-transmitting glass fibre cable has been another advance in endoscopy.

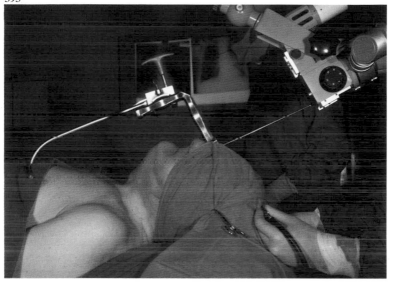

Tracheostomy

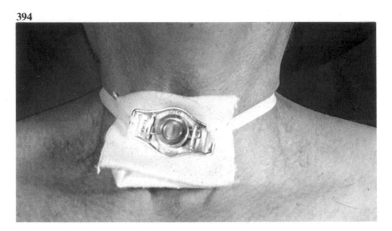

394 A patient after tracheostomy Obstruction of the larynx causes stridor and may necessitate a tracheostomy. Acute inflammatory conditions of the upper respiratory tract eg epiglottitis, or foreign bodies or neoplasms limiting the airway are the commonest causes of stridor.

Tracheostomy is also required for respiratory failure due to central depression of the respiratory centre eg strokes, barbiturate poisoning, head injury, poliomyelitis or tetanus. Multiple rib fractures or severe chest infections may require tracheostomy. Tracheostomy enables breathing to be controlled by an intermittent positive pressure respirator, and bronchial secretions can be removed with suction. A prolonged obstruction of the glottis may occur with juvenile papillomas, severe trauma to the larynx, or with bilateral cord palsies, and a permanent tracheostomy is necessary. A tracheostomy tube with a *speaking valve* allows air to enter during inspiration but closes on expiration so that air passes through the larynx for phonation.

Emergency tracheostomy may be a difficult operation, particularly under local anaesthetic when a general anaesthetic with intubation is not practical. An opening into the trachea through the cricothyroid membrane offers a simpler and more direct relief for upper respiratory tract obstruction.

395

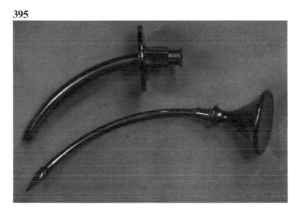

395 Cricothyrotomy cannula with trocar This instrument has been devised for emergency operations. A tracheostomy can be performed later when the emergency of the acute obstruction is past.

396 Tracheostomy Openings are usually made between the 2nd and 3rd tracheal rings. A 'higher' tracheostomy predisposes to stenosis of the larynx in the subglottic region. The airway is most accessible and superficial at the level of the cricothyroid membrane and in acute laryngeal obstruction an opening through this membrane will restore the airway. The **cricothyrotomy** opening is, however, for emergency and is temporary. Indwelling tubes at this site lead to subglottic stenosis of the larynx.

396

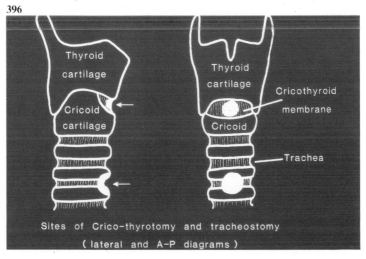

Sites of Crico-thyrotomy and tracheostomy
(lateral and A-P diagrams)

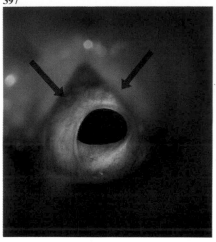

397 Subglottic stenosis Slightly hyperaemic cords can be seen in this patient with an area of ring-like stenosis below the vocal cords. This stenosis followed trauma, partly related to a road traffic accident in which the trachea was injured, and also related to a high tracheostomy through the first tracheal ring. Dilation is rarely effective for this type of cicatricial stenosis and excision of the stenotic area of the trachea with end-to-end anastomosis is necessary.

The hypopharynx and oesophagus

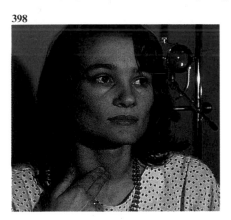

398 Globus pharyngeus This is a very common condition in which the patient, not infrequently a young girl, complains of a sensation of a lump in the throat. The site indicated is the cricoid region. In the history a helpful direct question is to ask whether the lump is most apparent on swallowing food, fluid or saliva: the patient with globus will consistently reply that saliva is the problem, and that the symptom occurs *between* meals.

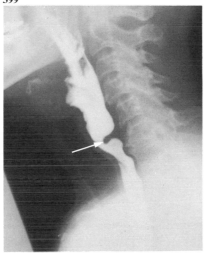

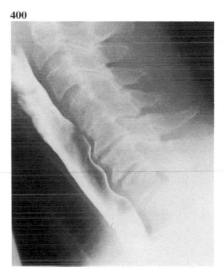

399, 400 Barium swallow Globus pharyngeus is a psychosomatic condition but there is demonstrable spasm of the cricopharyngeus on barium swallow, where the barium column is seen to be 'nipped' (**399**). Over-attention and concern by the patient perpetuates the spasm and reassurance and explanation is usually the only treatment required.

Globus pharyngeus does not necessarily occur in hysterics and globus hystericus is a misnomer. It is also a condition that calls for investigation, particularly in the older age group, when it may be the presenting symptom of disease in the oesophagus or stomach. Hiatus hernia and oesophageal reflux commonly cause cricopharyngeal spasm, and gastric ulcers and neoplasms may also present with globus. A barium swallow and meal is therefore an important investigation. Cervical osteoarthritis (**400, 401**) with marked changes in the region of the 6th cervical vertebra may also give rise to globus.

401

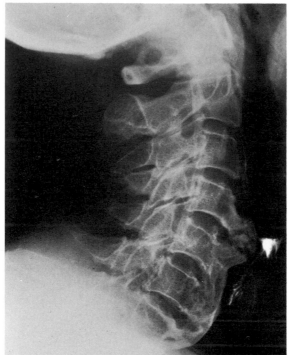

401 Cervical osteoarthritis Projection of cervical osteophytes into the post-cricoid region of the upper oesophagus causes cricopharyngeal spasm and the symptom of globus. In this X-ray gross osteophytes have caused 'nipping' of the barium by the cricopharyngeus muscle.

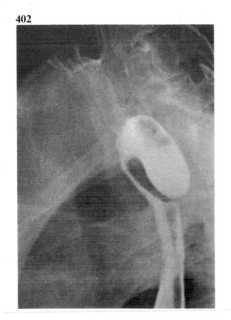 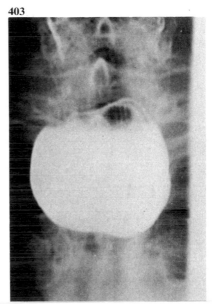

402, 403 Pharyngeal pouch This is a herniation of mucous membrane through the posterior fibres of the inferior constrictor muscle above the cricopharyngeus, usually occurring in old age. The defect predisposing to its development is a failure of co-ordinated relaxation of the cricopharyngeus on swallowing. A pouch is frequently associated with a hiatus hernia.

A small pouch causes no symptoms but when large, dysphagia develops, varying from slight to absolute, there is regurgitation of undigested food, and gurgling may be heard in the neck after eating, or a swelling may be seen, laterally in the neck, usually on the left. The pouch accumulates food, and spillage into the respiratory tract may cause coughing. A pouch may present with respiratory disease, either bronchitis, or apical fibrosis simulating tuberculosis, or as acute pulmonary infection—bronchitis, bronchopneumonia or a lung abscess.

The barium swallow is the only investigation required to confirm the diagnosis of a pharyngeal pouch.

If symptoms are marked, excision of the pouch via a neck incision is necessary. Rarely a carcinoma occurs within the lumen of a pharyngeal pouch.

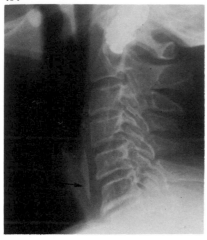

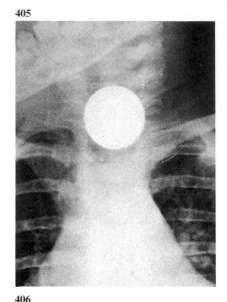

404–406 Foreign bodies in the oesophagus Foreign bodies such as bones, coins, pins, dentures and small toys, may impact in the upper third of the oesophagus. A history of possible foreign impaction must not be ignored for oesophageal perforation leads to cervical cellulitis and mediastinitis, which may be fatal. Air seen on X-ray behind the pharynx and oesophagus is diagnostic of a perforation. Persistent dysphagia, pain referred to the neck or back, pain on inspiration and fever all suggest a foreign body. Chest X-ray and X-ray of the neck are essential investigations, but even if negative, persistent symptoms are suspicious and oesophagoscopy is necessary. Coins, however, which pass the cricopharyngeus usually traverse the rest of the gut, and rarely require removal.

406

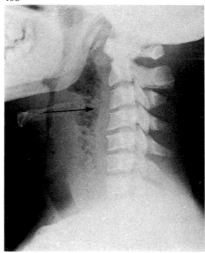

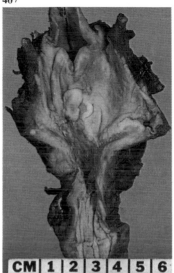

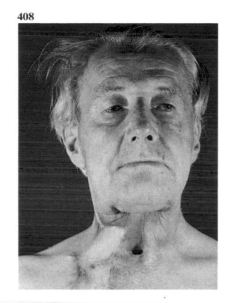

CM| 1 | 2 | 3 | 4 | 5 | 6

407, 408 Carcinoma of the pyriform fossa and upper oesophagus The presenting signs are dysphagia for solids, and pain, commonly referred to the ear. There is early metastasis to the cervical nodes. A carcinoma involving mainly the medial wall of the pyriform fossa causes hoarseness. The prognosis is not good, particularly with upper oesophageal carcinoma, whether treatment is with radiotherapy or surgery. Resection for these carcinomas involves a pharyngo laryngectomy and the replacement or reconstruction of the cervical oesophagus poses technical problems. Immediate replacement with stomach or colon mobilised and brought through the thorax and sutured to the pharynx are current techniques. The delayed use of neck and chest myocutaneous flaps is an alternative method of reconstruction. Microvascular surgical techniques have enabled immediate reconstruction with a section of the ileum and is a further option.

The Head and Neck

Salivary glands

409

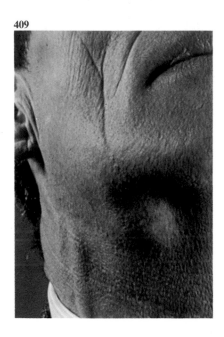

409 Submandibular calculus A calculus obstructing the submandibular duct causes painful and intermittent enlargement of the gland. The swelling occurs on eating and regresses slowly: secondary infection in the gland leads to persistent tender swelling of the gland.

The swelling in the submandibular triangle is visible and palpable *bimanually*, with one finger in the mouth.

410 Grossly enlarged submandibular gland This develops if an impacted calculus is ignored. A neoplasm of the submandibular gland is the differential diagnosis if the enlargement is persistent and there is no evidence of a calculus on X-ray. The nodular surface and the firm, non-tender character on palpation of this gland are also suggestive of a neoplasm, commonly a pleomorphic adenoma or adenoid cystic carcinoma. Mumps may also cause a tender submandibular gland swelling, and an enlarged lymph node in the submandibular triangle, secondary to dental infection, simulates gland involvement.

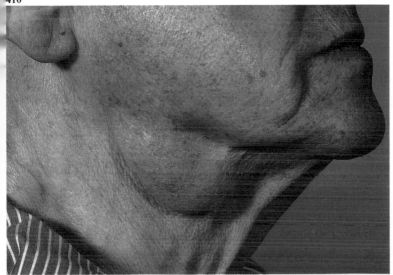

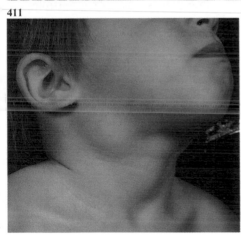

411 A tonsillar lymph node enlargement may be similar to an enlarged submandibular gland. This node is frequently palpable in children, being more conspicuous at times of tonsillar or upper respiratory tract infection, and the node, as in this case, may become very obvious. The node is soft and tender. Exact location of the site is important: it is posterior to the submandibular triangle at the angle of the mandible.

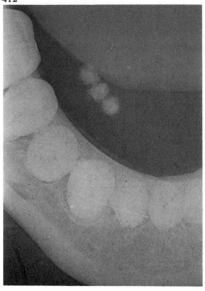

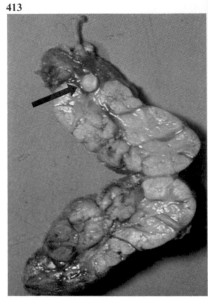

412 X-ray of the submandibular gland region demonstrating calculi in the duct.

413 Calculus impacted in the gland If the calculus is in the duct, removal by intra-oral incision is effective. If, however, the calculus is placed posteriorly in the duct or is impacted in the gland (as here) excision of the submandibular gland is required. Care is taken in this operation to preserve the mandibular branch of the facial nerve which crosses the submandibular triangle to supply the muscles of the angle of the mouth.

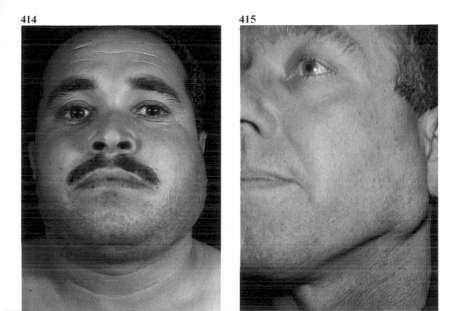

414, 415 Mixed parotid tumour (pleomorphic adenoma) These present as a firm smooth non-tender swelling. The growth is slow so the history may be long. The bulk of the parotid lies in the *neck* posterior to the ramus of the mandible, and parotid tumours do not usually cause predominantly facial swelling.

416   417

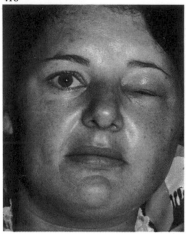 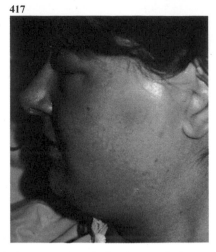

416, 417 Mumps Acute viral parotitis is a common infection and the diagnosis is usually obvious. Well-defined tender swelling of the parotid gland, first on one side and shortly after on the other, with associated trismus and malaise are characteristic. Mumps, however, can be deceptive when it remains unilateral and the swelling is not strictly confined to the parotid. In this case of mumps the swelling involved the side of the face causing lid and facial oedema. Unilateral total deafness is a not uncommon complication of mumps.

418

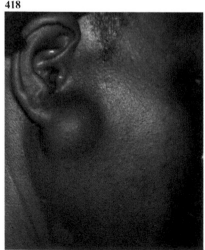

418 Sebaceous cyst A swelling in the parotid region, but *on the face* suggests another diagnosis: there is a small punctum on the swelling in this picture, diagnostic of a sebaceous cyst.

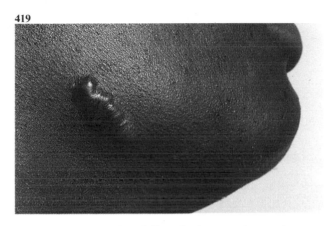

419

419 Sebaceous cyst on the face Minor lesions such as sebaceous cysts present a problem on the face when excision is needed: the scar may be obvious and unacceptable. Particular care, therefore, is needed to enucleate these cysts meticulously, through incisions made within the relaxed skin tension lines. It may also be necessary to 'break-up' the straight incision line so that it is less obvious. A keloid is a further concern particularly in the coloured and this followed excision of a sebaceous cyst in the upper neck.

420 Congenital hypertrophy of the masseter muscle Careful palpation follows observation of a swelling, and what appears as a parotid mass here is palpable as a congenital hypertrophy of the masseter muscle.

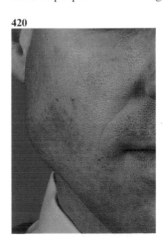

420

A softer swelling in the tail of the parotid may be an *adenolymphoma* (Warthin's tumour) a benign tumour of salivary gland tissue within a parotid lymph node. The pleomorphic adenoma is a low-grade malignant tumour, and is commonly in the superficial lobe of the parotid: treatment is superficial parotidectomy with preservation of the facial nerve. A soft parotid swelling with a short history and a partial or complete facial palsy is probably an adenoid cystic carcinoma or higher grade malignant tumour of the parotid gland requiring total parotidectomy with sacrifice of the facial nerve, and radio-therapy.

421

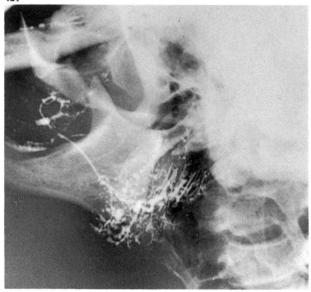

421 Sialectasis of the parotid gland This presents as intermittent episodes of painful swelling. Calculi in the parotid duct are uncommon and are not easily demonstrated on X-ray. An intra-oral view is necessary. A sialogram confirms sialectasis, and the punctate dilations of the parotid ducts are similar in appearance to bronchiectasis. The parotid swelling with sialectasis is often infrequent and mild and triggered by certain foods. There is no simple treatment and superficial parotidectomy is reserved for the rare, severe cases.

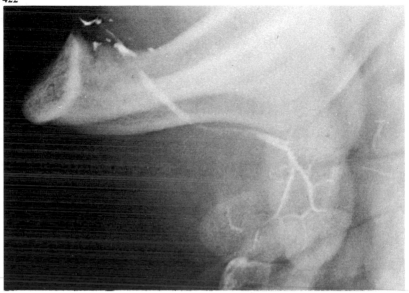

422 Normal submandibular sialogram The pattern of ducts not involved with sialectasis is demonstrated. A parotid sialogram is not difficult to perform for the duct orifice opposite the second upper molar tooth is obvious and can be made more apparent by massaging over the parotid gland, causing a visible flow of saliva. The submandibular duct orifice anteriorly in the floor of the mouth is not obvious; cannulation for sialography may be difficult.

Inflammatory neck swellings

Spread of dental infection must be remembered as a possible cause of inflammatory neck swelling.

423

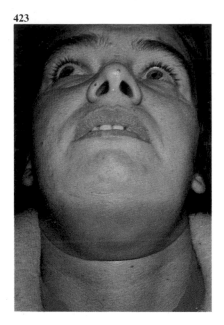

424

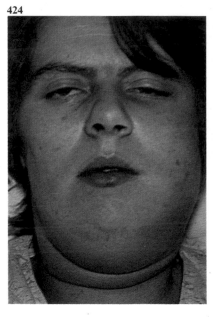

423 Ludwig's angina An indurated tender *midline* inflammation is characteristic of Ludwig's angina. Bimanual palpation reveals a characteristic woody firmness of the normally soft tissues of the floor of the mouth and this is an early sign. This acute infection may spread from the apices of the lower incisors and in this case followed extraction. In the pre-antibiotic era this condition was serious because spread of infection involved the larynx, and caused the acute onset of stridor. This complication is still to be remembered although extensive neck incisions to relieve pus under pressure are rarely necessary, and the response to intramuscular penicillin is good.

424 Cervical cellulitis may develop from a dental abscess in the lower molars and involve the neck laterally.

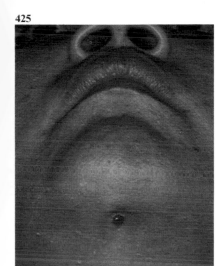

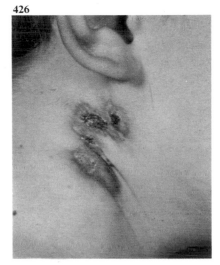

425 Submental sinus A chronic localised midline infection under the chin is probably a submental sinus. This recurrent mass of granulation tissue formed at the opening of a sinus leading to apical infection in a lower incisor.

426 Tuberculous cervical abscesses These are uncommon in countries where cattle are tuberculin-tested, for intake of infected milk is the usual cause. A chronic discharging neck abscess in the posterior triangle is characteristic of tuberculosis. Firm, non-tender nodes without sinus formation in the same site are also suggestive of tuberculosis. Chemotherapy alone usually fails to control this condition and excision of the nodes or chronic abscesses is required.

Midline neck swellings

427

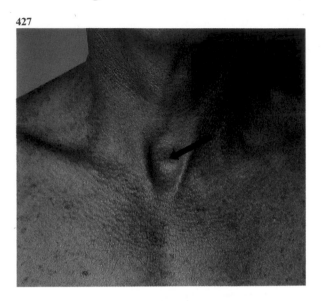

428

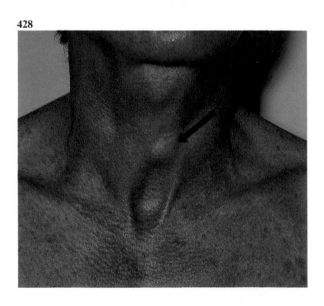

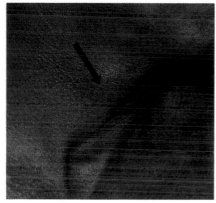

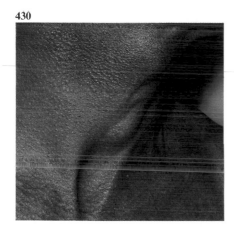

427–430 Thyroglossal cyst This is a midline neck swelling forming in the remnant of the thyroglossal tract. The swelling is commonly between the thyroid and hyoid but suprahyoid cysts also occur. The convexity of the hyoid bone and thyroid cartilage push the cyst to one side so it may not be strictly midline. The cyst moves on swallowing and on protrusion of the tongue. It may be non-tender or present with recurrent episodes of acute swelling and tenderness. Treatment is excision with removal of the body of the hyoid bone. Failure to excise the body of the hyoid predisposes to recurrence for the thyroglossal tract extends in a loop deep to the hyoid bone.

431

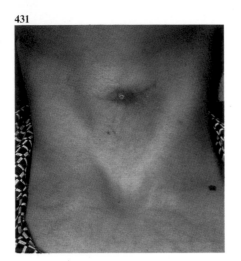

431 Thyroglossal cyst Excision of the cyst alone, without the tract and body of the hyoid bone leads to recurrence. The cyst remnant causes inflammation and discharge at the scar. This appearance is characteristic of an inadequately excised thyroglossal cyst.

432

433

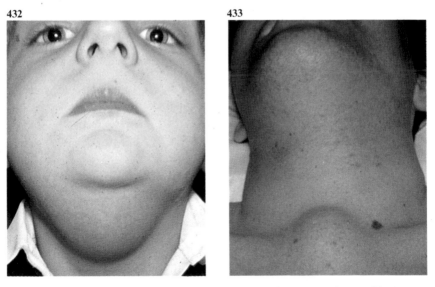

432, 433 Dermoids Midline neck swellings in the submandibular region (**432**) or suprasternal region (**433**) are commonly dermoids.

Lateral neck swellings

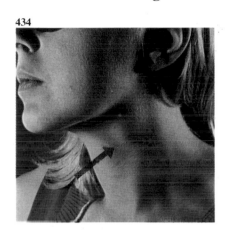

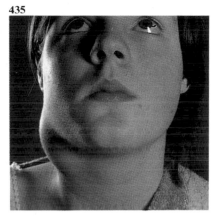

434–436 Branchial cyst This has a consistent site, is smooth and, if there is no secondary infection, is non-tender. It lies between the upper one-third and lower two-thirds of the anterior border of the sternomastoid and is deep to and partly concealed by this muscle (**436**). It can be large, therefore, by the time it presents. When excised the deep surface is found to be closely related to the internal

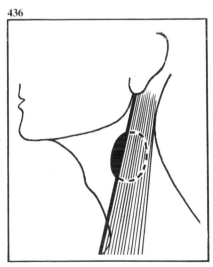

jugular vein. A metastatic lymph node from the thyroid, upper respiratory tract (eg nasopharynx), or postcricoid region, and swellings of neurogenous origin (chemo-dectomas, neurofibromas, neuroblastomas) are among the important differential diagnoses of a lateral neck swelling. The ubiquitous lipoma is also not uncommon in the neck, and in children the cystic hygroma is to be remembered. Hodgkin's disease also frequently presents with an enlarged cervical lymph node.

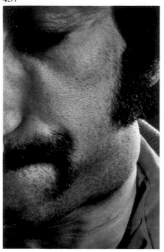

437 Laryngocele This is an unusual neck swelling that the patient can inflate with the Valsalva manoeuvre. It is an enlargement of the laryngeal ventricle into the neck between the hyoid and thyroid cartilage. It tends to occur in musicians who play wind instruments, or glass blowers. Infection may develop in laryngoceles (a **pyolaryngocele**), and presents as an acute neck swelling often with hoarseness and stridor.

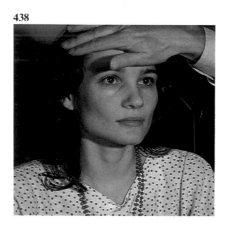

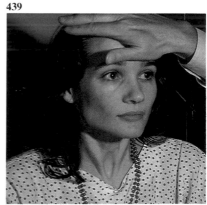

438–440 Test for accessory cranial nerve function (XI) The sterno-mastoid muscle is supplied by the accessory nerve. If the patient is asked to press the forehead against the examiner's hand, the sternal attachments of the muscle stand out. When the XIth cranial nerve is inactive, the sternal head on the side of the lesion remains flat (**440**).

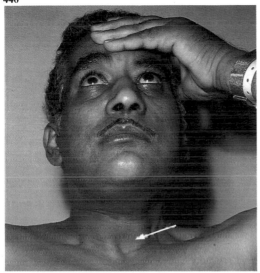

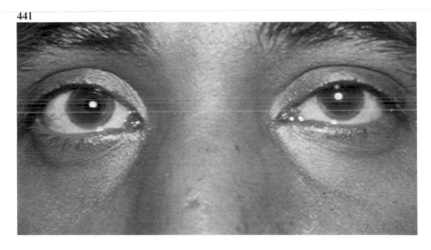

441 Horner's syndrome Pressure on the sympathetic nerve trunk in the neck, particularly by malignant disease, causes changes in the eye. Ptosis, with a small pupil, is apparent in the patient's left eye: this is also associated with an enophthalmos and a lack of sweating. With a cervical swelling examination should exclude Horner's syndrome.

Index

Figures in **bold** type refer to
illustrations; other figures refer to
page numbers.